GURTNER
DETROIT
HEALTH
DEPT

VALUES IN SEXUALITY

A New Approach
to Sex Education

VALUES IN SEXUALITY

A New Approach to Sex Education

**ELEANOR S. MORRISON
& MILA UNDERHILL PRICE**

HART PUBLISHING COMPANY, INC.
NEW YORK CITY

CONTENTS

CONTENTS

VALUES IN SEXUALITY

A New Approach to Sex Education

INTRODUCTION

IS A NEW STYLE OF EDUCATION for mature sexuality possible? We believe so. The teaching and learning designs contained in this book have been successfully utilized over a number of years with students at Michigan State University. Yet this is not the traditional method of teaching a university course (or an adult-education class or a high-school course). Often, the assumption underlying the traditional method is that education comprises a one-way flow of information from expert to learner. Certainly, accurate information is essential, but it is not sufficient. There are many kinds of information, and many ways of acquiring information. The assumption underlying the approach in this book about human sexuality is that *affective responses to sexual issues are as important as cognitive ones.*

The fundamental issues relating to human sexuality encompass the personal value system, life style, self-image, communication mode, and philosophy about how persons in relationship act toward each other. Any course of study in sex education must deal with all of these individual realities, in addition to information or external facts, if the learner is to live as a responsible citizen and sexual being in our pluralistic society.

The late Isadore Rubin pointed out that although it is impossible to achieve consensus about sexual values, it is urgent that we deal truthfully and critically with the variety of sexual value systems. Rubin urged that the very same at-

9

titudes that are unquestionably the foundation of sound scholarship and pedagogy—critical intelligence, a respect for truth, the right of individuals to self-determination—be applied to the taboo-laden area of education about human sexuality.[1]

"In teaching politics and government," Rubin wrote, "we do not feel the need to indoctrinate all students into being members of one or another political party. Rather, we try to teach them the skills and attitudes which they require to make intelligent choices as adults when faced with a changing world and an array of alternatives."[2]

Teaching human sexuality can take the same approach, and this is the one used in this book. Perhaps in no other area of human behavior is there so much diversity in attitudes, feelings, and actions as there is in the area of sexuality. *Values in Sexuality* is designed to provide students with a variety of exercises and discussion activities that will enable them to take a close and critical look at their more-often-than-not hidden feelings about sex. To examine these feelings through frank and open discussion, students meet with their peers of both sexes, in small groups of from six to eight persons.

The teaching/learning designs presented here are primarily interaction exercises, with the purpose of increasing self-awareness, catalyzing individual thought, critical self-assessment, and—through a confrontation with diversity—value clarification. There are no right or wrong responses to the problems posed. The only "examinations" are the continual self-examination which occurs in the process of group

---

1   Isadore Rubin, "Transition in Sex Values—Implications for the Education of Adolescents," *Journal of Marriage and the Family,* May 1965, pp. 185-189.
2   op cit., p. 187.

interaction. Clearly, the outcome of this process is difficult to measure quantitatively. However, we confidently anticipate that the interaction exercises in this book will yield qualitative gains in terms of:

1. Freedom of individuals to examine and talk about sexual issues;

2. Clarity about one's personal values vis-à-vis the conflicting value systems of others;

3. Sensitivity to the importance of plain, direct talk about sex;

4. Conscious awareness of the destructive potentialities inherent in some cultural and interpersonal expressions of sexuality;

5. Appreciation for oneself, one's body, one's sexuality.

While the approach in this book precludes endorsement or condemnation of any particular point of view with regard to sexual codes, there are certain assumptions underlying these teaching/learning approaches. They include the following:

1. Human sexuality is a function of the *total* personality, and is not limited to genital or reproductive processes.

2. Most people need a structure which permits them to explore and discuss sexual issues.

3. Interpersonal communication is a crucial component of

healthy sexuality. Sex is not something men do to women, nor is it a guessing game in which each partner tries to "psych out" the other, rather than indicate personal preferences and pleasures.

4. Education for human sexuality is a life-long process which is not concluded with a sex-education course. The continuing process looks like this:

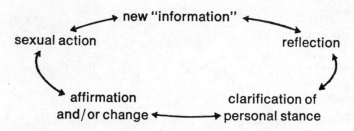

5. "Learning about human sexuality must include a personal focus—reflecting on, and grappling with, one's own experiences, knowledge, convictions, and values—tested against the experience, attitudes, beliefs, insights, and values of persons from different cultural and family traditions . . . To learn about human sexuality is to deal not only with information about gonads, orgasm, and coitus but also with a kind of personal knowledge about oneself and one's sexual role."[3]

Since this book focuses primarily on an educative process, it must assume a background of content. For a list of recommended content resources, see the back of the book.

Because of the rapid obsolescence of information related to public issues involving sexuality, the texts and exercises presented in this book may be supplemented by

3 Eleanor S. Morrison and Borosage, Vera, *Human Sexuality: Contemporary Perspectives,* National Press Books, Palo Alto, California, 1973, pp. x, xi.

films, by readings in current events (court cases on abortion, pornography, etc.), and by lecture presentations from such organizations as the Gay Liberation Movement, Right to Life, etc.).

As the teacher gains experience in using the interaction designs which follow, he will easily see ways of adapting these methods for use with such issues as pornography, prostitution, venereal disease, censorship, abortion, illegitimacy, sex laws, sex and racism, population control.

A note about the setting for, and use of, these teaching/learning designs: Although the material was originated for use in a course at Michigan State University, the material has also been utilized in a wide variety of other settings—for example, in workshops to provide in-service training for teachers, clergymen, counselors and paraprofessionals in the helping professions; in consciousness-raising groups; in family camps; in church groups; and in parent groups.

To make the most effective use of these designs, the participants should meet in a room or rooms large enough to permit the group to be broken up into sub-groups of from two to eight persons. Members of the sub-groups should be able to talk together without undue interference from other sub-groups.

Specific directions for implementation of this program, including exposition of goals, procedures, and materials, are given. It is hoped that teachers may be inspired to enhance and supplement these suggestions in ways that will be applicable to their particular groups.

ELEANOR S. MORRISON
MILA UNDERHILL PRICE
East Lansing, Michigan

GROUP-BUILDING ACTIVITIES

SUBJECT: *The Name Game*

MATERIALS NEEDED: None.

TIME REQUIRED: 5-10 minutes for a group of eight.

OBJECTIVES:

To emphasize the importance of knowing and using people's names as a means of indicating that each person is valued.

To build a sense of group cohesion and morale.

To introduce members to each other, and to provide practice in remembering names.

RATIONALE:

Although people vary in the importance they attach to their names, most people would rather be called by their own names than be addressed in some general way. One of the prerequisites to effective group functioning—especially if the group is to tackle an area beset with as many taboos as human sexuality—is that the members begin to feel they can trust each other. Using names in personal address is a minimal first step in this process of getting to know each other, and building a sense of community.

PROCEDURE:

1. Form a circle.

2. Give the following directions:

    "We will be talking about all sorts of things which concern us personally. When I talk to people, I like to be identified as *(first name)*, not as some nameless person who happens to be speaking. It is important to me that people know and remember my name, and use it when they are talking to me. You may not feel as strongly about this, but it probably makes you feel good when other people remember your name and use it.

    "To help us remember each other's names, I will start by saying my name. Then the person to my right will give the name that he/she prefers being called, and will repeat my name. We will continue around the circle with each person in turn giving his/her name and repeating the names of those who went before."

3. After all have introduced themselves, change the seating arrangement and practice again.

4. This game may be played at the beginning of the first two group meetings.

※   ※   ※

SUBJECT: *Obstacles to Discussing Sexual Issues*

MATERIALS NEEDED:

A large sheet of newsprint for each group of six.
A felt-tip pen or marker for each group.

TIME REQUIRED: 20-30 minutes.

OBJECTIVES:

To bring to the surface the anxieties and fears which impede discussion of sexuality.

To begin the trust-building process.

RATIONALE:

Discovering that the anxiety and discomfort provoked by a course on sexuality is shared by other members of the group is helpful in dissipating these fears. This sharing experience marks the beginning of the trust-building process, which is so important for this kind of group.

The way the task is stated allows persons to generalize difficulties they may not feel ready to admit are their own. If an individual can discuss the general discomfort felt in the group (without specifically identifying it as their own) they may feel freer to take the next step, and share a feeling of their own.

PROCEDURE:

1. Instruct the participants to form groups of six, and to be sure that not everybody in the group already knows each other.

2. Pass out paper and pen or marker to each group. Then give these directions:

    "In this course, we will be exploring issues related to human sexuality. Before we begin, discuss with the members in your group the following question: 'What makes it difficult to talk about sexual issues in a group like this?'

    "List on the newsprint all the comments your group comes up with. Place an asterisk by those which most of you view as primary difficulties."

3. Give a few minutes warning when time is almost up. Instruct the groups to post their lists on the wall when they are finished.

4. When all the lists are posted, allow time for reading the lists. Perhaps one person in each group will read its list aloud. If other members of that group care to make additional comments, they should be encouraged to do so.

5. After all the lists have been read, ask the people to comment on what similarities they see in the lists.

※   ※   ※

SUBJECT: *Getting Acquainted*

MATERIALS NEEDED: None.

TIME REQUIRED: 5-15 minutes.

OBJECTIVES:

To begin building a group identity by sharing data about self with the group.

To begin the practice of self-disclosure at a relatively safe level.

To encourage each person in the group to feel he/she has an important contribution to make.

RATIONALE:

One of the important groundwork activities that enables a group to function as a group is the sharing of personal information. When people know a little about each other, know a little about what to expect from each other, and become familiar with the personal experiences out of which people speak and act, they may feel more trust in the group and therefore be more ready to speak of intimate, important matters.

In this activity, people are free to reveal whatever they feel comfortable letting the group know. There is no pressure to be intimate, to tell all. When the subject matter is sex, people need the reassurance that they are in charge of what they talk about—that there will be no coercion or pressure to move beyond what they themselves perceive to be appropriate. This is especially true at the ice-breaking stage in a group's life.

PROCEDURE:

1. Instruct students to break into groups of six.

2. When groups have formed, give the following directions:

   "Each of us is a unique person, with a unique background, a unique perception of the world. Getting to know another person—just one other person—is a very complicated process. And we are, hopefully, going to try to get to know five to seven other persons.

   "Think about yourself, and about how you can let your group get acquainted with you. If you had to choose only two things that most accurately describe you, what would they be? Take a few seconds to think about how you would describe yourself. Then each of you tell the other people in your group two things that are most characteristic of you."

2b. *Alternative procedure*

   Provide each person in the group with a sheet of construction paper and a felt-tip pen or crayon. Ask each to choose two personal characteristics, and then draw pictures to illustrate these characteristics. Each individual pins or tapes the paper to his/her chest and, without talking, looks at the representations of the others in the group. Afterwards, all talk about each other's self-portraits.

2c.   *Alternative procedure*

Each person share: "Two things I do when I feel comfortable in a group."

"Two things I do when I feel uncomfortable in a group."

2d.   *Alternative procedure*

Each person share: "Two things that turn me on."

"Two things that turn me off."

※   ※   ※

SUBJECT: *Touching*

MATERIALS NEEDED:

Strong tables (strong enough to hold the combined weight of six people), or smallish areas on the floor marked off by masking tape.
Blackboard, chart, or overhead transparency.
Pencils and paper.

TIME REQUIRED: 5-15 minutes.

OBJECTIVES:

To contribute to a sense of group identity through fun-and-games activity.

To provide an experience of enforced closeness on the basis of which the group can share personal feelings about touching and closeness.

To encourage the sharing of personal feelings, preferences, convictions.

RATIONALE:

Providing an activity the group can share is helpful in building a sense of "we-ness." The fun-and-games atmosphere reduces self-consciousness and inhibition, while enabling persons to express their feelings about physical closeness. The participants may feel "safer" about disclosing their attitudes before other members of the group than they would without the legitimizing structure of the game.

This activity evokes good-natured interchange, which adds to the sense of groupness and enhances morale.

PROCEDURE:

1. Instruct participants to form groups of six.

2. Introduce exercise:

    "The next activity will help you get acquainted with the people in your group in a different way. Please clear the tops of your tables (presuming you are using tables; if the floor is being used, adjust instructions accordingly).

    "This is a kind of contest to see how well your group functions in relation to the other groups here. Here are the rules of the contest. All members of each group are to climb onto the top of the group's table. No arms, legs, or clothing may hang over the edge of the table, and no one may stand on the table. I will announce which group is first to carry out these instructions correctly. Keep your positions until I call time.

"Ready? Go."

3. Look at each group. Indicate where a leg, or a hand, or whatever, is visible over the edge of the table. As each group perfects its table-top posture, call its number and point to it. *Remind the members to hold their positions.*

4. Continue:

"Now, become aware of the fact that you are touching people. Look at the positions of all the members of your group. Are you back-to-back? Face-to-face? Which parts of your bodies are touching? Which aren't? O.K., you can get down now, and talk among yourselves about the exercise."

5. When each group untangles to discuss the exercise, here are some possible areas for them to explore (the list may be presented on a chart or overhead):

   a. How did you feel while we were doing this exercise?

   b. How do you usually feel about close physical touching?

   c. Were you conscious of trying not to touch people in certain ways?

   d. Do you feel closer to or further away from the members of your group? Why?

☼   ☼   ☼

SUBJECT: *Stop-Action: How're We Doing?*

MATERIALS NEEDED:

Printed or verbal assessment questions.

TIME REQUIRED: 5-45 minutes (depending on group).

OBJECTIVES:

To have the group focus on the *process* of their group interaction.

To have the participants discover patterns of interaction which are characteristic of their particular group.

To allow people to express their satisfaction or frustration with the way the group is operating.

RATIONALE:

The *content* of a group discussion or interaction is only one part of the group life. The other part is the *way* that the content is being dealt with. Often, this aspect of how a group functions is ignored.

By deliberately stopping a discussion in midstream and asking people to pay attention to the dynamics of their group, they become more conscious of the various processes by which a group functions well.

When people feel they can influence the direction of an

enterprise, they are likely to have more zest for that activity. The stop-action reflection period allows participants to express their perceptions about how the group is functioning, and thus influence the future course of the group.

PROCEDURE:

1. Stop-action group assessment can be accomplished in different ways:

    a. Instructions can be given orally to all groups at the same time by interrupting the discussion with a predetermined signal—a buzzer, flicking the lights, etc.

    b. Written instructions can be placed in envelopes which are given to each group. One person would open the envelope and read to the group the instructions they are to respond to. This procedure can be used at a random time in the group discussion, or at a time when the group seems to be in special need of looking at their process.

1. On the next page are examples of the kind of stop-action instructions that may be given (orally or written). When the group has completed its stop-action discussion, the members may return to the topic they were discussing earlier. In addition to taking part in the stop-action discussion, each member of the group may do his or her own evaluation of the group discussion process. Forms for such evaluation may be found on pages 27-28.

Stop-Action Instructions

I. Stop what you are doing, and take a look at how your group is listening.

  a. Are you hearing from *all* members of the group? *If not, why not?*

  b. Are people *listening* to what other people say, or are they talking past each other?

  c. Are you giving verbal and nonverbal evidence to the speaker that he/she is being heard?

II. Are you respecting each other's views?

  a. How willing are you, as individuals, to take (and defend) a position that seems to be unpopular with the group?
  b. Are you "giving in" to avoid conflict? Why, or why not?
  c. Are you listening to other people's views with an open mind?
  d. Is it possible to be honest in responding to these questions?

Group-Assessment Samples

I. *How Well Are We Listening?*

Using the scale below, rate your group's ability to listen to others with understanding.

Level 1: Continues with own agenda, ignoring the person speaking.

Level 2: Responds, but with own ideas or feelings, not acknowledging what was said.

Level 3: Gives nonverbal evidence (eye contact, head nod, etc.) that what was said was being heard.

Level 4: Able to hear and repeat the speaker's words to speaker's satisfaction.

Level 5: Able to relay speaker's feelings—as well as words— back to speaker in a nonjudgmental way.

Most people in the group responded at level _____.

A few people in the group responded at level _____.

No people in the group responded at level _____.

I feel I generally responded at level _____.

II. *Where Am I in This Group?*

Assess the validity of the statements below from 1-5, 1 being "very much" and 5 being "very little."

———— I feel I can really talk in this group about things that matter to me.

———— I feel I am an effective part of the group.

———— I feel free and able to use the group as a sounding board for my attitudes and feelings.

III. *How Well Is My Group Functioning?*

Using the scale below, record your choice of ranking in the blank opposite each statement.

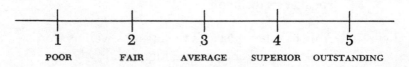

1	2	3	4	5
POOR	FAIR	AVERAGE	SUPERIOR	OUTSTANDING

1. Participation by all members. ————.

2. Diversity of values and ideas, freely expressed. ————.

3. Esprit de corps, sense of "groupness." ————.

4. Warmth, acceptance, trust among members. ————.

5. Willingness to initiate activity, interest in trying something new. ————.

Total ————.

PHYSIOLOGY

THE TRADITIONAL APPROACH to sex education has been to focus on the "facts of life," which have generally been understood to mean the physiology of reproduction. The assumption has been that once these anatomical matters have been discussed, the subject of human sexuality has been covered.

While a basic understanding of the physiological basis of sexual response is extremely important, many other issues are more important in an individual's development of a mature sexuality.

Nevertheless, the authors have found it useful to begin with the physiology of sex. This seems a low-threat way of helping people begin to deal with their own sexuality. An initial concentration on physiological data enables students to ask questions and to express confusion, things they may be reluctant to do in regard to their *feelings* about sex.

In working with community groups, we have found the use of the true-false sex-information survey helpful for some of the same reasons. It seems easier for people to begin to talk about "intellectual" sexual matters than about "emotional" ones. However, if the group of students is to meet for only one or two sessions, we bypass the physiological exercises, since personal-value issues are of much higher priority.

SUBJECT: *Vocabulary Brainstorming*

MATERIALS NEEDED:

Overhead projector (optional).
Transparency naming the "four languages of sexuality" (see step 2 of PROCEDURE).
Chart or transparency with discussion questions.
Microphone (if room and group are large).

TIME REQUIRED: 30-60 minutes.

OBJECTIVES:

To make it easier to talk about sex by using a variety of sexual words in a mixed group.

To build a team spirit and to energize the individual group members.

To provide a structure for sharing and reflecting on feelings about the explicit vocabulary used.

RATIONALE:

Students often refer to a sexual activity or organ as "it," "doing it," etc. This exercise legitimizes and encourages the use of more explicit vocabulary—scientific, or direct, or "street vocabulary."

Working together on a task that calls for quickness and competition helps to lower inhibitions and to heighten group cohesiveness.

It is often difficult for individuals to talk about their feelings unless the structure explicity gives them permission.

PROCEDURE:

1. Form groups of 6 to 8 persons.

2. Introduce the exercise by saying:

     "For any discussion, one must learn the language of the subject matter. A discussion of sexuality is no exception. However, sexuality can be discussed in at least four different languages:

     a. "The language of science: words such as cervix or coitus, designed for precision.

     b. "Childhood language: words such as weewee or number 2, designed to hide embarrassment and circumvent confrontation.

     c. "Street language: words such as fuck or cock, designed to describe vigorously and sometimes demeaningly.

     d. "Common discourse: words or phrases such as making love or having sex, designed to communicate information plainly and uneuphemistically."

For reinforcement, put a transparency listing the four languages on the overhead projector.

3. Leader continues:

     "We are now going to do some brainstorming. To brainstorm means to generate as many words as possible without any discussion or evaluation. The primary purpose of this procedure is to increase our ease in talking about sex in a sexually mixed group. I will say a sexual word, and as soon as it is given, each group is to brainstorm and write down all the synonyms for that word, using any or all of the four languages of sex.

"Choose one person to be the recorder in your group, to write down the words as quickly as you say them.

"When I call time you are to stop. Then we'll check and see which group won, that is, had the most synonyms.

"The first word is *penis*."

4.   Leader calls time after 2 to 3 minutes, and asks each recorder to count the synonyms the group has brainstormed. After the winning group has been determined, ask the recorder of that group to read off his list of synonyms for *penis*. Ask the other groups to add words of their own which were not mentioned by the winners.

5.   Leader continues:

"Next word, *intercourse*."

Increase allotted time slightly.
Repeat step 4 after each word. Generate synonyms for such words as vagina, breast, masturbation, homosexuality, etc.

6.   When you feel your students have engaged in a sufficient amount of brainstorming, place on the overhead (or chart) the following questions for the students to discuss in their groups:

Questions for Group Discussion

1. How did you feel about doing this exercise?
   Did your feelings change as the exercise progressed?

2. Did you find it difficult to say some words?
   What made it difficult?

3. Did the presence of the opposite sex inhibit you?
   If so, was that more true with some words than with others?

4. Were there any surprises for you in this exercise?

5. Are there any general patterns to the synonyms for any of the brainstorming words? Did you notice, for instance, the "weapon" overtone of some of the words, and the "put-down" implied in some?

※   ※   ※

SUBJECT: *Vocabulary Brainstorming* (alternate design)

MATERIALS NEEDED:

Large sheets of newsprint.
Several felt-tip pens for each sheet of newsprint.

TIME REQUIRED: 30-60 minutes.

PROCEDURE:

1. On each large sheet of newsprint leader writes one word or phrase, such as:

PENIS	MASTURBATION
VAGINA	V.D.
INTERCOURSE	BREAST
MALE HOMOSEXUAL	FEMALE HOMOSEXUAL

2. The sheets are scattered around the floor or posted on walls, several pens by each sheet.

3. Individuals walk around and write whatever synonyms they think of under each heading, at the same time circling those words on the list they have never heard of.

4. When this task is completed, form groups of 4 to 6 persons.

5. Each group examine one chart at a time, and talk about the meanings of circled words.

In 1972-73, the authors compiled the following data on three stimulus words their students used in the Vocabulary Brainstorming exercise. In two separate classes, a total of 23 groups—each composed of 5 to 7 persons—students drew up lists of synonyms for *penis, vagina,* and *intercourse.* The groups included both men and women students, with a higher number of women in every group.

Those synonyms appearing on fewer than five lists are not included in the tabulations below.

I PENIS

WORD	FREQUENCY	WORD	FREQUENCY
Cock	21	Dingdong	9
Dick	20	Hot Dog	9
Prick	20	Pecker	7
Peter	18	Gun	7
Rod	17	Phallus	7
Weewee	15	Pee-pee	6
Thing	14	Pistol	6
Shaft	14	Organ	6
Ding-a-ling	11	Joint	5
Dink	10	Schmuck	5
Wiener	10	Meat	5
Stick	9		

II   VAGINA

WORD	FREQUENCY	WORD	FREQUENCY
Cunt	21	Honey Pot	11
Box	21	Cave	8
Hole	20	Lips	7
Pussy	20	Snatch	7
Cherry	14	Privates	6
Down There	13	Clitoris	6
Twat	13	Beaver	5

III   INTERCOURSE

WORD	FREQUENCY	WORD	FREQUENCY
Fuck	22	Score	10
Screw	22	Sleep With	8
Lay	20	Mess Around	8
Do It	20	Go to Bed	8
Make It	17	Have Sex	8
Ball	19	Make Babies	7
Make it	17	Knock Up	7
Hump	14	Roll in the Hay	7
Fornicate	14	Know	7
Go All the Way	14	Mate	7
Get It On	13	Pump	6
Copulate	12	Get Down	6
Coitus	12	Carnal Knowledge	6
Bang	10	Mount	5
Rape	10	Procreate	5

※   ※   ※

SUBJECT: *Sex-Information Survey (true-false)*

MATERIALS NEEDED:

A copy of sex-information survey (pages 39-44) for each person.

TIME REQUIRED: 20-30 minutes.

OBJECTIVES:

To inform students of their own level of sex information.

To dispel myths of human sexuality.

To legitimize asking questions about the physiological aspects of sex.

To give the leader(s) a rough measure of the students' level of sexual knowledge.

RATIONALE:

If students sort out their areas of ignorance and areas of knowledge at the beginning of the course, this increased self-awareness can motivate them to learn more.

Sharing questions and uncertainties about such relatively objective material as is contained here may demonstrate to the students that ignorance is no disgrace. In turn, this will make it easier for students to air more personal questions and confusions at a later time.

The more the leader(s) knows about the level of knowledge of his group, the more he/she is able to meet the needs of the particular students.

PROCEDURE:

1. Form groups of 6. Hand out *Sex-Information Survey* on page 39, and give these instructions:

    "This is a true-false survey to help you discover what you know about human sexuality. Please complete it individually, without consultation."

2. When all have completed the survey, indicate that every third proposition is true (#3, #6, #9, etc.). Each student is to correct his/her own paper.

3. Ask each group to tally up the questions missed most frequently, and to discuss those which the group members are most interested in, or those which were most often missed.

Sex-Information Survey

	TRUE	FALSE

1. Sex is an intense, high-pressure drive which forces the sexually mature person to seek immediate gratification. If such gratification is impossible, serious physical and emotional effects may result.   ____ ____

2. A woman must reach orgasm in order to conceive.   ____ ____

3. Both men and women experience nocturnal orgasms.   ____ ____

4. Husband and wife must experience simultaneous orgasms for conception to occur.   ____ ____

5. Simultaneous orgasms are an indication of optimal sexual interaction.   ____ ____

6. Women may have gonorrhea without any obvious symptoms.   ____ ____

7. Women are not often capable of multiple orgasms.   ____ ____

8. A woman is absolutely safe from conception if sexual intercourse occurs during menstruation.   ____ ____

TRUE   FALSE

9. Recent studies of homosexuality have not solved the question of its cause.   ____   ____

10. Easy penile penetration without pain or bleeding is a sign of nonvirginity.   ____   ____

11. There is a safe period in the menstrual cycle during which it is impossible for conception to occur, and this is the period immediately following menstruation.   ____   ____

12. Alcohol can be a common cause of temporary impotence.   ____   ____

13. Menstrual cramps and pain most frequently have a physiological cause.   ____   ____

14. The sex drives of men and women show a significant decrease at about the age of 35 to 40 years.   ____   ____

15. Prenatal biochemical influences are very important in sexual development.   ____   ____

16. An orgasm for a woman achieved by vaginal penetration is more satisfying and requires more maturity than orgasm resulting from direct clitoral stimulation.   ____   ____

17. Sexual intercourse should ordinarily be avoided during menstruation.   ____   ____

	TRUE	FALSE

18. Lack of girl playmates in childhood has little causal relationship to male homosexuality. ____ ____

19. Women lose interest in sexual activity after the menopause or after a hysterectomy. ____ ____

20. For health reasons, it is generally unwise to have intercourse during the last six weeks of pregnancy. ____ ____

21. Active sex play during childhood or adolescence indicates normal growth and curiosity. ____ ____

22. Laws governing sexual behavior are relatively rare but well-enforced. ____ ____

23. Black people have a stronger sex drive than white people. ____ ____

24. Sexual attitudes of children are more strongly molded by attitudes of significant adults than by pornography, erotic TV and movies, or excessive sex play. ____ ____

25. The size of a man's penis bears a direct relationship to his potency and virility. ____ ____

26. A large penis is necessary for a woman's sexual gratification during coitus. ____ ____

TRUE   FALSE

27. Sexual dysfunction is much more frequently a matter of psychological fac-
tors than physiological disturbance.   ____   ____

28. Research indicates that the main sexual
outlet of the typical male college fresh-
man or sophomore tends to occur with
a girl he loves and may someday marry.   ____   ____

29. An imbalance of hormones causes homosexuality.   ____   ____

30. Drugs have more direct relationship to
sexual fantasies than to heightened sexual proficiency.   ____   ____

31. College girls are more likely to have premarital coitus than are girls of the same
age who do not attend college.   ____   ____

32. Homosexuals can ordinarily be identified by certain mannerisms or physical
characteristics.   ____   ____

33. Premature male climax can be delayed
by the woman squeezing the penis when
excitement intensifies.   ____   ____

34. Homosexual men are more creative than
heterosexual men.   ____   ____

TRUE   FALSE

35. Married men of low educational achievement have an increasing incidence of extramarital sexual intercourse between their twenties and thirties.   ____   ____

36. The sex assigned to a child and the way he or she is reared are the primary determinants of psychological maleness and femaleness, thus overcoming chromosomal factors.   ____   ____

37. Generally speaking, women who have a strong sex drive, who come to climax easily, and are capable of multiple orgasms are nymphomaniacs.   ____   ____

38. In the middle and later years, sexual activity is markedly decreased because of physiological changes.   ____   ____

39. The sex drive of a woman may be as powerful as that of a man, especially in the middle years.   ____   ____

40. The most inappropriate time for a child to be exposed to sex education is during the preschool years.   ____   ____

41. Masturbation can result in almost total depletion of seminal fluid.   ____   ____

TRUE   FALSE

42. Genitalia of both sexes originate from the same cell mass.   _____   _____

43. In a case of infertility, the woman is almost always the defective partner.   _____   _____

44. Sperm that have been deposited in the vagina one or two days prior to ovulation are capable of fertilizing the egg.   _____   _____

45. The sixth week of pregnancy (four weeks after a missed period) is the earliest point at which a physician can determine with any reliability that a woman is pregnant.   _____   _____

46. In lesbian couples, one of the two always assumes a "male" or "butch" role.   _____   _____

47. Vasectomy is an easily reversible form of contraception.   _____   _____

48. Infants are capable of having orgasms.   _____   _____

49. College men generally have about the same amount, or more, of premarital coital experience than do men of lower educational achievement—and at an earlier age.   _____   _____

๑๑   ๑๑   ๑๑

SUBJECT: *Physiology Definition*

MATERIALS NEEDED:

A set of definition sheets (see pages 47-50) for every two people in the class.
Pencils.

TIME REQUIRED: 30 minutes.

OBJECTIVES:

To review physiological terms relating to sex.

To practice the use of sexual vocabulary in the group.

To legitimize areas of ignorance about physiology and to provide a comfortable setting in which ignorance may be revealed.

RATIONALE:

Using a direct, uneuphemistic vocabulary not only facilitates discussion, but also makes the participants more at ease about the subject matter.

The social pressure to appear "all-knowing" about sex makes it difficult for many to admit ignorance. This exercise legitimizes such an admission.

PROCEDURE:

1. Introduce the exercise by explaining the RATIONALE.

2. Instruct students to form pairs, with a member of the opposite sex if possible.

3. Direct each pair to take one set of definition sheets and find a place in the room where they can fill in the answers without disturbance from others in the group. In completing the sheets, the pair should share their knowledge, noting those answers about which they are unsure.

4. Returning to groups when finished, students compare answers (see page 51) with other group members, giving special attention to those answers on which pairs disagreed. Leader should emphasize the importance of using the actual words, rather than numbers or letters, during steps 3 and 4 of this procedure. (Say "clitoris" rather than "#12.")

Physiology Definition Sheet I

Put the proper number in the blank.

1. Premature ejaculation	5. Abortion	10. Gonorrhea
2. Foreplay	6. Sterility	11. Menopause
3. Impotence	7. Vaginismus	12. Puberty
4. Erection	8. Menarche	13. Ejaculation
	9. Miscarriage	14. Chancre

A. _____ Inability in the male to achieve erection.

B. _____ Inability to produce offspring.

C. _____ Spontaneous expulsion of the fetus from the uterus at any time between the onset of the fourth month to the end of the sixth month of pregnancy.

D. _____ Premature expulsion from the uterus of a fertilized ovum, an embryo, or a nonviable fetus.

E. _____ Onset of menstruation in girls, occurring in late puberty.

F. _____ Period of cessation of menstruation, usually between ages 45 and 53.

G. _____ Stiffening and enlargement of the penis or clitoris as blood engorges the spongy tissue during sexual arousal.

H. _____   Strong muscular contractions within the vagina, preventing entry of the penis in intercourse.

I. _____   Communicable venereal disease with minimal symptoms in the woman.

J. _____   Period of physical growth at which human beings become capable of procreation.

K. _____   Emission of seminal fluid, usually at orgasm.

L. _____   Sore or ulcer that is the first symptom of syphilis.

M. _____   Ejaculation prior to, just at, or immediately after insertion of the penis into the vagina.

N. _____   Caressing and other activity designed to arouse sexual excitement prior to intercourse.

Physiology Definition Sheet II

Put the proper number in the blank. Definitions may be matched with more than one term.

1.	Seminal vesicles	12.	Clitoris
2.	Scrotum	13.	Gonad
3.	Uterus	14.	Vas deferens
4.	Amnion	15.	Circumcision
5.	Semen	16.	Ovum
6.	Placenta	17.	Labia majora
7.	Sperm	18.	Egg
8.	Afterbirth	19.	Glans penis
9.	Bag of waters	20.	Fallopian tube
10.	Ovary	21.	Vagina
11.	Testes	22.	Vulva

A. _____ Pouch containing the testicles.

B. _____ Pear-shaped organ in the female, where the fetus grows until birth.

C. _____ An organ of spongy blood cells by which the baby is attached to the lining of the uterus, and through which the fetus is fed and wastes are eliminated.

D. _____ The membrane forming the closed sac of fluid in which the unborn child is immersed within the uterus.

E. _____ Whitish fluid ejaculated by the male at climax, containing male sex cells (in fertile males).

F. _____ Mature reproductive cells of the male which are capable of fertilizing the female ovum.

G. _____ Female reproductive cell, which after fertilization begins developing into an embryo.

H. _____ Cone-shaped head of the male sex organ.

I. _____ Egg-conducting tube that extends from each ovary to the uterus.

J. _____ Canal from the external sex organs of the female to the cervix.

K. _____ Removal of the foreskin from the penis.

L. _____ Female reproductive gland.

M. _____ Male sex glands.

N. _____ A small, highly sensitive female sex organ located where the inner folds of the vulva meet.

O. _____ External sex organs of the female.

P. _____ Two pouches in the male, opening into the sperm ducts.

Q. _____ Sperm ducts in males leading from epididymus to the seminal vesicles and the urethra.

R. _____ Outer pair of lips of female external genitals.

ANSWERS

Sheet I

A.	3	H.	7
B.	6	I.	10
C.	9	J.	12
D.	5	K.	13
E.	8	L.	14
F.	11	M.	1
G.	4	N.	2

Sheet II

A.	2	J.	21
B.	3	K.	15
C.	6, 8	L.	10, 13
D.	4, 9	M.	11, 13
E.	5	N.	12
F.	7	O.	22
G.	16, 18	P.	1
H.	19	Q.	14
I.	20	R.	17

SUBJECT: *Group Drawing of Female and Male Reproductive Anatomy*

MATERIALS NEEDED:

Large sheets of paper.
Pencils.
A chart or transparency with an accurate drawing of the female and the male reproductive organs.
A chart or transparency listing the organs to be included in the student drawing.

TIME REQUIRED: 30-40 minutes.

OBJECTIVES:

To indicate the basic knowledge students have about human anatomy (and the gaps in that knowledge).

To provide a setting in which ignorance about physiology may be revealed without shame.

To provide an opportunity to work as a group on a task.

RATIONALE:

The primary purpose of this exercise is to provide a relaxed, "non-academic" means of reviewing the basic sexual physiology. Many students feel they learned all there was to know about physiology in junior high school, but this exercise may reveal how hazy their knowledge of anatomy really is.

PROCEDURE:

1.   Give the following instructions:

"Break up into groups of four to six persons, with men and women in each group. Take a large sheet of paper and pencils for your group. (This exercise may be conducted on an individual basis rather than as a group.)

"Since we are talking about sexuality, it might be helpful to discover how accurately we know the structure of the sex organs. Each group is to make a cross-sectional drawing of the female anatomy and one of the male anatomy. Include in your drawings all the parts I have listed here. See how well you can do on your own, without referring to any books. Pool your group resources. You have 15 minutes to complete both drawings."

MALE ANATOMY	FEMALE ANATOMY
Penis	Vagina
Scrotum	Uterus
Testes	Ovary
Vas deferens	Fallopian tubes
Prostate	Clitoris
Glans penis	Urethra
Urethra	Bladder
Bladder	Labia majora
	Labia minora
	Cervix

2.   When the allotted time is up, give the following instructions:

"I will now place on the overhead accurate drawings

of the female and male reproductive organs. Check your
drawings carefully and correct them. Talk about inaccu-
racies in your drawings."

(A transparency can be made from illustrations in
standard texts, such as McCary, James, *Human Sexuality*,
Van Nostrand, New York.)

※   ※   ※

SUBJECT: *Venereal Disease Information Survey (true-*
false)

MATERIALS NEEDED:

An information survey for each person.
Pencils.
Resource persons (public health or other) to answer ques-
tions.

TIME REQUIRED: 15-30 minutes.

OBJECTIVES:

To provide some accurate information about the nature of
venereal disease.

To legitimize admission of ignorance about V.D.

PROCEDURE:

1. Have students form small groups of five to seven.

2. Hand out the V.D. Information Survey presented on pages 56-57, and give the following instructions:

    "This is a true-false survey to help you discover what you know about venereal disease. Please complete it individually without consultation. As you complete the survey, check those statements which you would like to question or discuss in the group."

3. After everyone has completed the sheet, display the answers below on a chart or transparency:

1.	False	8.	True	14.	False
2.	False	9.	False	15.	True
3.	True	10.	False	16.	True
4.	False	11.	True	17.	False
5.	True	12.	False	18.	False
6.	False	13.	False	19.	False
7.	True				

4. When students have finished their answers ask them to discuss the questions which were most often missed by the members of the group.

Venereal Disease

	TRUE	FALSE
1. V.D. is not a significant risk to me if I limit my sexual contacts to the university community.	____	____
2. Like most infections, V.D. will either get worse or go away.	____	____
3. Men are more likely to know if they have V.D. than are women.	____	____
4. If you are a minor and are treated for V.D., your parents are likely to be informed.	____	____
5. Women may have gonorrhea without symptoms until complications arise.	____	____
6. The symptoms of gonorrhea are sometimes undetected by the male while those of syphilis are painful enough to be noticed.	____	____
7. The complications of gonorrhea are sometimes sterility, while those of syphilis are sometimes brain damage or death.	____	____
8. People who have V.D. are asked (in confidence) to name their sexual contacts.	____	____

		TRUE	FALSE

9. V.D. is not a possible result of homo-sexual contacts. ____ ____

10. Self-administered doses of oral peni-cilin are usually sufficient to cure gon-orrhea or syphilis. ____ ____

11. The incidence of gonorrhea is twice that of syphilis. ____ ____

12. Getting an annual blood test is usually sufficient to detect the presence of V.D. ____ ____

13. V.D. is not a possible result of oral-gen-ital contact. ____ ____

14. There are no primary symptoms of syph-ilis in either men or women. ____ ____

15. The primary symptoms of gonorrhea in a male is a thick, creamy discharge from the penis. ____ ____

16. "Crabs" is another sexually transmitted problem. ____ ____

17. Another name for syphilis is "clap." ____ ____

18. V.D. can be transmitted through toilet seats and dirty glasses. ____ ____

19. A condom is 100% protection against syphilis or gonorrhea. ____ ____

PSYCHOSEXUAL DEVELOPMENT

SUBJECT: *Sharing of Childhood Memories*

MATERIALS NEEDED:

Chart on which to write cues for discussion, or an overhead projector and transparency.

TIME REQUIRED: Variable—one could spend an hour or an entire day on this exercise.

OBJECTIVES:

To identify and express to others some personal experiences and feelings related to sexuality.

To increase awareness of how personal attitudes about sexuality develop.

To discover the universality of most sexual feelings and experiences.

To practice the skill of self-disclosure within a small group.

To identify how one's present attitudes and feelings toward sex are related or unrelated to early experience.

RATIONALE:

Virtually all people tend to view their personal feelings and experiences as unique. Through this sharing of past experiences, many participants are greatly relieved to discover that their sexual feelings and experiences are shared by others. This discovery reduces the individual's sense of isolation and guilt, and allows him/her to be more self-accepting.

Many persons seem to need a structure of this kind to grant them "permission" to share.

Because childhood memories are from the distant past, the sharing process is less threatening. Also, this narrow focus on childhood allows for private sorting out, making it easier for individuals to decide what they want to share, and what they do not. In this approach, it is not likely that anyone will feel compelled to share more than he/she is ready to share.

There is a tendency to equate self-disclosure with "telling all," "baring one's soul." In this exercise, the leader stresses that self-disclosure also includes sharing what you are feeling right now, even if that means stating a preference not to talk about a given issue at this time.

Through this sharing process, individuals often are able to recall experiences and feelings which they had forgotten or blocked out. One person's experience triggers the recall of another person's experiences, which may greatly enrich the individual insights of each member of the group.

PROCEDURE:

1. Instruct participants to form trios, with a female and a

male in each. Suggest that they not group with close
friends or partners from earlier discussion groups, if possible. Have each trio find a private space and make themselves comfortable, facing one another.

2. In introducing this exercise, it is helpful to give persons
    the option of not sharing, while suggesting that they
    may want to mentally note the feelings that may come
    to mind, so these can be dealt with later, privately.

3. Introduce the exercise:

"Today we are going to share childhood memories
and experiences of sexuality. I will introduce each topic
of discussion, and then blink the lights when it is time
to move on to a new area. Some of you may not be ready
to move on, while others may be ready before I give the
signal. Therefore, in addition to introducing each topic,
I will place the topics on this chart (overhead); this will
allow you to be more flexible with your time.

"In learning about human sexuality, the biological
aspects of sex and reproduction are certainly important.
But equally significant are the affective aspects — the
attitudes, feelings, taboos which we privately have about
sexuality. These are learned in two places—most signif-
icantly in the family, and secondarily in the street, from
our peers as we are growing up.

"Today we are going to share some of these experiences and memories. You may find that you can't recall
any experiences in a particular area; you may have
blocked out experiences and feelings, perhaps because
you learned they were bad, or dirty. You may also find
that someone else's sharing triggers off a flood of memories you had forgotten about.

"One of the purposes of this exercise is to increase your awareness of how you felt about sexuality as a child, what you learned from your parents. This in turn will help you to understand your present feelings, and also to clarify what attitudes you wish to change, or wish not to pass on to others.

"You may discover there are some experiences you prefer not to share with your group. Do not hesitate to say so. Share only what you wish to share. You may want to let your partners know you are reticent about speaking, even though you have decided to share. That, too, is a kind of self-disclosure—sharing how you feel at the moment. For personal reflection later, you may want to note those actions and statements which make you feel ill at ease in your group."

4. In this section of the procedure, it is wise to move quickly through the first three topics, and increase the time allotment as the exercise develops.

Before sharing, students should take a few minutes for reflection. Leader says: "Reflect, then share."

  a. "What feelings do you recall about being a girl or being a boy, and how did you feel toward children of the opposite sex (envy, disdain)? Did your parents expect different things of you than they expected of your sisters (brothers)? If so, how did you feel about that?"

Five minute pause.

  b. "What were your family patterns in regard to: talk about sex; nudity; physical expression of affection?"

Seven minute pause.

c.   "What memories do you have of sex play as a child? If your parents were aware of it, what did they say or do? What were your feelings about sex play?"

Increase time for sharing on these subjects, allowing a few minutes for reflection before each one:

d.   "When did you first become aware of your parents' sexuality? What feelings did you have?

e.   "What did you learn about sex from peers of the same sex as yourself? What from peers of the opposite sex? What feelings did you have about these events and/or information?

f.   "What memories do you have of same-sex experimentation and exploration in late childhood and early adolescence? What feelings did you have about these experiences?

g.   "What memories do you have of: approaching adolescence; menstruation; wet dreams; awareness of sexual feelings; body development (or lack of it)? What were your feelings at the time?

h.   "What are your memories of the first time you were kissed or touched by a member of the opposite sex? What do you recall about your first love? Your first serious sexual involvement?

i.   "What was your most pleasurable or memorable sexual experience? This experience may be alone, relating to your sense of yourself as a man or a woman; or it may be with another (not necessarily a genital experience).

j.   "In what ways is your 'personal history' related or unrelated to your present feelings about your own sexuality?

k.   "What have you learned about your sexual development through this exercise? How do you feel about this experience?"

Topic k. may be discussed among the entire class or in the trio, depending upon the size and make-up of the class. If the class functions well as an ensemble, we have found it beneficial for the students to come together for a final sharing.

NOTE: Some of these topics may not be appropriate for certain groups. For example, "h" and "i" may be too close to the experience of some young people for them to want to share. Also, time limitations may require that some topics be omitted.

※   ※   ※

SUBJECT: *Drawing Yourself As an Adolescent*

MATERIALS NEEDED:

A large sheet of newsprint for each participant.
Crayons, or felt-tip pens, or paints for drawing.

TIME REQUIRED: One hour minimum for a group of six.

OBJECTIVES:

To increase awareness of how each person felt about himself/
herself as an adolescent.

To identify personal sexual experiences and concerns common to all adolescents.

To discover how those experiences and concerns have helped
shape one's present self-concept.

RATIONALE:

Drawing a visual image of yourself as an adolescent brings
to consciousness the feelings you had then. Often, persons
include in a drawing significant details of which they aren't
consciously aware. Other group members often see meanings
in a picture which help clarify what the artist felt during
that stage.

It is helpful to discover the universality of feelings about one's
own sexual development. This sharing experience builds trust
in the group and in oneself. It also frequently reduces uncer-

tainties and guilt feelings that individuals have long been carrying inside themselves.

This reflection-and-sharing experience often provides the participants with new data which help them to understand some of their present attitudes toward sex.

PROCEDURE:

1. Instruct the participants to form groups of six, with females and males in each group. Pass out a large piece of paper (12″ x 18″ newsprint, for instance) and drawing instruments to each group.

2. Leader instructs:

    "Close your eyes and reflect for a few minutes on what you looked like and what you felt like as an adolescent. What other persons were important to you then? Whom did you spend time with? How did you feel about yourself?

    "Take a few moments to remember yourself at age 14 or 15, and then without talking to anyone, draw a picture of yourself on the paper. You may want to include in the picture other people or objects which were important to you then.

    "Remember, this is not an art class; drawing ability is not important for this exercise."

3. After 10 minutes have passed, suggest that the students finish their drawings in the next two minutes.

    "Take turns in sharing your picture with your group. Tell them how you felt about your body as an adolescent, how you felt about yourself. Explain your picture. The others in the group should share with the artist what they see in the picture."

Let the group know how much time they have for this exercise, so they can divide that time in six, so each person has a chance to share his/her picture.

SEX ROLES

SUBJECT: *Personal Reflection and Self-Portrait*

MATERIALS NEEDED:

One large sheet of newsprint per person.
Crayons, felt-tip pens, or paints.

TIME REQUIRED: 30-45 minutes.

OBJECTIVES:

To explore personal feelings about one's own sex role.

To share personal feelings and perceptions of self with a small group.

To learn what other persons in the group see in your self-picture.

RATIONALE:

Drawing facilitates a self-discovery and disclosure which is not possible through verbal interaction. The choice of colors, shapes and lines often expresses perceptions the artist is not consciously aware of.

67

Using the picture as the focus makes it easier to share with group members how one sees oneself. This exercise provides a "safe" framework for group members to share responses to the picture, and for the artist to accept or reject their interpretations.

PROCEDURE:

1. Form groups of six.

2. Say the following:

> "Our focus today is on yourself as masculine or feminine. As a preparation for today's session, I invite you to 'center down' on yourself, on your own experience. Some people find it easier to center down if they close their eyes and relax—that's up to you."
> *Pause.*

> "Think of the reality that is *you* here in this room. It is *you* inhabiting that body. And think of that body of yours. Stand back and look at it—as if you were looking at yourself nude in a mirror. What is your body like?"
> *Pause.*

> "Think about your body as if you were discovering it for the first time—the curves, the flat and rounded surfaces, the angles, the hair, the texture and color of the skin, the general outline. What pleases you? What disturbs you?"
> *Pause.*

> "Has your body made a difference in the way you have conducted your life as a man or a woman? How?"
> *Pause.*

> "Think about your genitals and how they look—or feel. How do your feelings about your genitals relate to

your feelings about yourself as a man or a woman?"
Pause.

"Think about those aspects of your personality—your temperament, your spirit, if you will—which are unique to you. How would you characterize yourself?"
Pause.

"Now stand off from yourself and watch yourself walk down the street. Watch yourself approach another person—man or woman. What do you do? How do you look as you approach yet another person? Watch yourself as you approach. Stay with those images."
Pause.

"All of these and much more are who you are—you in particular—and there is no carbon copy anywhere. Who are You?"
Pause.

3. Give drawing instructions:

"Take the next few minutes and translate some of these thoughts and feelings and images into a self-picture, using the paper and crayons (pens, paints). This is not an art class. Simply portray, in whatever form you want to, how you see yourself as a man or a woman."

4. Allow five to ten minutes for drawing, then give the following instructions:

"When all group members have finished their drawings, take turns sharing your pictures. One person will hold up his/her drawing and remain silent while the other five in the group tell what they see in the picture. Remember that what anyone says is only a hunch based on what is seen. You are free to reject any interpretation that does not seem accurate.

"When this process is finished, the person who drew the picture should share what the picture means to him/her."

5. At the completion of the exercise, you may want to suggest that people save their pictures, and repeat this exercise at home to see how differently they perceive themselves at different times.

6. The leader may want to provide some guides to interpreting the pictures:
    a. The use of particular colors—"what does that color symbolize to you?"
    b. The significance of closed and open symbols—circles, dotted lines, broken circles, etc.
    c. The significance of the kinds of lines used—curves, angles, arrows, free-form, etc.

7. Another dimension of self-image and role differentiation emerges if each participant draws a second picture of himself/herself as the opposite sex, and then explores his/her feelings related to the two pictures.

※   ※   ※

SUBJECT: *Advantages and Disadvantages*

MATERIALS NEEDED:

Large sheets of newsprint, to be marked off as a chart (see page 75).

A dark-inked felt-tip pen for each group.
Chairs for "fishbowl" section of exercise, steps 6-9 (you
may elect to sit on floor).

TIME REQUIRED: 60-90 minutes.

OBJECTIVES:

To increase awareness of the advantages and disadvantages
of cultural sex-role expectations for people of the opposite sex.

To explore and clarify with students of the same sex perceptions and feelings about the roles society forces upon those
of the opposite sex.

To engage in a total class experience of verbal sharing.

To talk about what it is to be a man or a woman, in the presence of the opposite sex group, but without rebuttal from
them.

RATIONALE:

Through exploring the positive and negative aspects of sex
roles, students are able to see the "flip side"—that for every
advantage enjoyed by the opposite sex there may be disadvantages. This realization will enable students to be more
empathic toward the opposite sex, and to be less simplistic
in their analysis of opposite-sex behavior.

Verbal sharing can assist a person in clarifying his/her own viewpoint, and in understanding how other people differ in their perceptions.

Individuals often want to know how other persons beside the ones in their group feel about a given topic; an occasional total class experience allows for this, and provides an opportunity for more diverse viewpoints to be expressed.

Verbal sharing with no opportunity for the listener to respond allows persons to listen more carefully and less defensively.

PROCEDURE:

1. Introduce exercise:

    "Today we are going to explore some of the advantages and disadvantages of being a man or a woman. For most of the time, we will be working in same-sex groups. The women's groups will be thinking about what it's like to be a man, and vice versa."

2. Form into same-sex groups of six to nine members.

3. Direct students to look at the chart or overhead transparency you have prepared. It should look like the model on page 75. Then say to the students:

    "Men's groups, take a sheet of newsprint and mark it off in the same way as the chart is divided. After you have written in the two headings at the top, write the word *woman* in the two blanks at the top heading. Women's groups, prepare your sheets in the same way, and write the word *man* in those two blanks.

"Now, in your separate groups, you are to list as many advantages and disadvantages as you can think of. List only items which *most* people in your group agree to and are serious about."

4. Allow 10-20 minutes for this process in same-sex groupings. Give a warning five minutes before you are ready to call time.

5. When the first group appears finished, then give next set of directions:

"When you have completed both columns of the sheet to the satisfaction of all in your group, exchange lists with a group composed of the opposite sex.

"Read the list of the opposite sex. Discuss in your same-sex group how you feel about their perceptions regarding the pluses and minuses of being a member of your sex. Which of their observations does your group agree with? Where do you disagree? Are there different reactions within your own group to these perceptions? Explore them."

6. Allow five to fifteen minutes, then say:

"Now we are going to have an opportunity to hear how people feel about their *own* sex role, about the advantages and disadvantages they experience as men or women.

"Each group choose _____ person(s) to participate with other members of the same sex in this discussion. These representatives will sit together in the center of the room, while the other students observe them and listen to their feelings and perceptions. Because the participants are encircled by silent observers, this process is called fishbowling." (Anywhere between five and eight persons of the same sex may occupy the fishbowl.)

7. Make a circle of chairs in the center of the room, leaving two chairs vacant.

    "Will the representatives come to the center? We will flip a coin to see whether the men or the women talk first."

    After the coin flip, say:

    "There are two vacant chairs in the circle. If any of the rest of the students of the same sex as those within the fishbowl want to say something, they may move into these chairs. After you have said your piece, please vacate the chair so someone else can occupy it.
    "The persons in the fishbowl are the speaking members of the discussion. The opposite sex is to remain silent during the fishbowl discussion."

8. In fishbowl discussion, persons tell how they feel about their own sex roles. Time allotted may be varied.

9. Reverse—have opposite sex form fishbowl and proceed as before.

Disadvantages of Being a ———	Advantages of Being a ———

SUBJECT: *How Do You Really Feel About Sex Roles?*

MATERIALS NEEDED:

Alternative I *(individual):* 56 statements for each person
(see page 83); tally sheet for each person (see 89); pencils.
Alternative II *(group):* large writing surface or overhead
projector; large room; 3 signs—AGREE, DISAGREE, NEUTRAL;
sufficient colored slips (four colors) for size of group; tally
sheet for each person; pencils.

TIME REQUIRED: 60-75 minutes.

OBJECTIVES:

To identify and clarify the attitudes of individuals toward
sex roles.

To discover patterns and consistency (or lack thereof) in
one's personal view of men's and women's roles in our society.

To increase awareness of the different ways one could view
male and female roles; to shed light on the options for individuals.

RATIONALE:

Individuals frequently resist being explicit about what they
believe. This forced-choice exercise pushes them to choose
between alternatives, and thus enables them to discover
where they really stand on particular issues related to sex
roles.

Often, people aren't aware that there are other ways than their own of viewing sex roles. Awareness of diversity is a first step toward the possibility of change and mature personal choice.

PROCEDURE: Alternative I *(individual)*

1. Form groups of six. Pass out to students a copy of the preference-sort survey presented on pages 83-88. Read the directions at the top of the sheet.

2. Introduce exercise:

    "Today, each of you is going to sort out what you believe about the roles of men and women. This exercise will be only a rough measure of what you feel, but it should·help clarify what you believe to be generally true about men and women. It is important that you place each slip not where you think you should put it, but rather where the slip will represent what you believe and value personally. Be honest with yourself. The directions are written out on top of the first page."

3. Allow 10-20 minutes for the sorting process, then say:

    "When you have finished, turn to the scoring sheet (see page 89). Before you tally up your score, look at the four different categories listed at the top. Mark which one you think you'll be highest in, which second highest. Now tally up your score as directed and see how accurately you guessed. Don't show anyone your tally sheet."

4. Allow five to ten minutes for tallying, then say:

    "Has everyone finished? If not, I'll give you a few

more minutes before the next set of directions."

5.   Offer this procedure as a possible group activity:

"When everyone in your group has completed the tally, those of you who wish to do so may take this time to receive feedback from your group members on how they see you in relation to these attitudes.

"If you volunteer to receive feedback, don't tell anyone how you scored. Each person will tell you what categories they would place you in. Jot that down. Does it jibe with your self-perception and/or the scoring sheet? If not, you may wish to ask the group members to give examples of your behavior in the group that caused them to categorize you in the way they did.

"Remember, if what you hear doesn't fit, you are free to reject it. Be sure to limit your time so that each person who wants to receive feedback can do so.

"When you are giving feedback, check yourself for tone of voice and word selection. See if you can give feedback without being judgmental. Be particularly aware of this when you are placing a person in an attitude category you feel very negative about."

6.   When the time is up, give the next set of directions:

"Use the remainder of the time to discuss issues which have emerged as being most troublesome to you, or areas about which there is most diversity of opinion in the group. Examine how others in the group view the male and female roles, and what effect their views may have on their behavior. How do views different from your own make you feel? A particularly useful way to generate discussion is to compare the slips you each put in pile #1 and pile #7."

PROCEDURE: Alternative II *(group)*

Arrangement of room and materials:

People will be moving about the room in this exercise. In three different parts of the room, place signs: AGREE, DIS-AGREE, NEUTRAL. At each sign, there will be numbered slips in four colors, in sufficient quantity for your group (if there are 30 people involved in the exercise, then you need 30 slips of each color at each sign).

Slips at the AGREE sign will be marked with a *3.*
Slips at the NEUTRAL sign will be marked with a *2.*
Slips at the DISAGREE sign will be marked with a *1.*

The slips are color-coded to the categories on the tally sheet:

> Old masculinist—pink.
> New masculinist—yellow.
> Old feminist—green.
> New feminist—white.

1.   Give instructions:

"Today, each of us is going to sort out what we believe about the nature of men and women, and the roles that society imposes upon them. This exercise will be only a rough measure of what you feel, but it should help clarify what you believe to be generally true about men and women.

"Posted around the room you see three signs: AGREE, DISAGREE, and NEUTRAL. I will read a statement from the center of the room. If you agree with the statement, go to the AGREE table and pick up a slip of the color I designate. If you disagree, go to the

DISAGREE table and pick up a slip. If you are neutral, go to the NEUTRAL table. Trust your gut reaction, what you *really* feel rather than what you may think you *should* feel. Be honest with yourself—that way you'll learn the most about yourself."

2. Read the first statement, which falls in the "new masculinist" category, and instruct the students to move to the appropriate table and pick up a yellow slip. The color to select for each slip is indicated in the margin opposite each statement.

3. Continue reading the statements. It might be helpful to say:

"Resist the temptation to move where your friends move. It might be easier for you to close your eyes as I read the slip, make your decision, and then move at once to the table of your choice. Be aware of how you feel when you're at a table by yourself or with only a few others, and everyone else is at another table. Is it hard to stick with your choice? Do you wish you had gone somewhere else so you wouldn't be conspicuous?"

4. If there seem to be significant patterns of movement within the entire group, you may wish to call attention to these patterns.

5. When you have read all 56 statements, instruct the students to return to their groups. Then read, or place on the overhead projector, the following four classification areas and give a brief description of each category. (See top of scoring sheet on page 89.)

Old masculinist
New masculinist
Old feminist
New feminist

6. Instruct:

"Each person write down which category you think you will be in." It might be helpful to remind the students that these four classifications are rough designations, not precise descriptions.

7. Place on overhead projector or chart, or simply read aloud the color code for each category.

Old masculinist: pink
New masculinist: yellow
Old feminist: green
New feminist: white

8. Then say:

"You are to sort the slips you have collected. Put all the slips of one color together. Record the numbers on the slips of each color, and total them up. You should have four totals. The higher the score in any one color, the closer you are to the position that color symbolizes."

9. After everyone has tallied up, continue:

"Those of you who wish to do so may take this time to receive feedback from your group members on how they see you in relation to these four attitudes.

"If you volunteer to receive feedback, don't tell anyone how you scored. Each person will tell you what category or categories they would place you in. Jot that down. Does it jibe with your self-perception and/or your tally? If not, you may wish to ask the group members to give examples of your behavior in the group that caused them to categorize you in the way they did.

"Remember, if what you hear doesn't fit, you are free to reject it. Be sure to limit your time so that each person who wants to receive feedback will be able to do so.

"When you are giving feedback, check yourself for tone of voice and word selection. See if you can give feedback without being judgmental. Be particularly aware of this when you are placing a person in an attitude category you feel very negative about."

10. As a final word, say:

"Use the rest of the time to talk about how you feel about your score. Does it surprise you? Does it make you feel comfortable or uncomfortable?"

Preference Sorting:
Men's and Women's Roles

DIRECTIONS: Tear statements apart, one statement to a slip of paper. Sort the slips into seven piles according to the scale below. On each slip, write the number of the statement. When you are finished, compute your score by following directions on the scoring sheet.

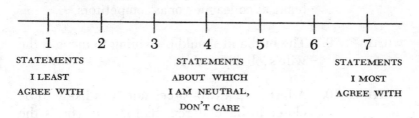

| 1 | 2 | 3 | 4 | 5 | 6 | 7 |

STATEMENTS
I LEAST
AGREE WITH

STATEMENTS
ABOUT WHICH
I AM NEUTRAL,
DON'T CARE

STATEMENTS
I MOST
AGREE WITH

YELLOW   1.   A career for a married woman is most appropriate after her children are grown.

YELLOW   2.   A woman may be employed, but should not compete with her husband for professional success.

GREEN   3.   A woman can best achieve full self-development by ignoring men and the system men have built.

YELLOW   4.   Women are better suited to work for men than men are suited to work for women—in making things run smoothly and efficiently with quiet assistance.

GREEN   5. The world can be much more efficiently run by women than by men.

WHITE   6. Alimony should be abolished.

YELLOW   7. It is a good idea for a woman to marry someone in the same field of work—in order to be a helpmate.

GREEN   8. If a woman marries, it is a good idea to marry someone in her field—in order to work as a team, as colleagues, or as competitors.

WHITE   9. The husband should be willing to move if the wife's job demands it.

WHITE   10. A father in a two-career family is likely to be closer to his children than is one who is the sole breadwinner.

GREEN   11. Men, because they are more subject to heart attacks and ulcers, and because they feel a need always to be in an authoritative position, are less equipped for difficult responsibilities than women.

WHITE   12. Women should be able to have abortion on demand.

YELLOW 13. Women are inherently more intuitive and empathic than men.

YELLOW 14. Women have special talents unique to their sex that should be better utilized.

YELLOW   15. A woman should be free to pursue whatever interest or vocation she pleases, providing it does not inconvenience her husband.

PINK   16. Women's natural work is in the home, but men should now and then assist them with their work.

GREEN   17. It is not society or the "system," but men who oppress women.

PINK   18. Women are instinctively maternal and nurturing.

PINK   19. Women should be educated, but not strive to become powerful or influential in public activity.

YELLOW   20. Women's most useful work in the world is to do the idealistic, community-minded things often neglected by men.

YELLOW   21. Women should be free to pursue many avenues of endeavor because modern men need women who are interesting, flexible, and capable.

WHITE   22. Sex roles are obsolete, and we should move toward desexregation so that eventually there are no "female" or "male" roles.

GREEN   23. Women can and should try to be like men.

GREEN   24. The enemy of women is men.

PINK   25. Girls should be raised in such a way that they will be proud to say that their sole vocation is wife and mother.

GREEN   26. Women should "wear the pants."

PINK   27. A woman's best job cannot be salaried—keeping a man happy.

WHITE   28. Women as well as men should be liable to the draft.

WHITE   29. Girls should be free to ask for a date, and to initiate sexual relationships.

PINK   30. Much as women would like to be good scientists, first and foremost they want and need to be mothers and companions to men.

GREEN   31. A woman would necessarily make a better President than would a man.

PINK   32. A woman cannot physically, emotionally, or psychologically do the work men do.

GREEN   33. It is better to be single than to be subordinate to a man.

GREEN   34. Women are superior to men in every way.

PINK   35. The trend toward desexualization in clothes, jobs, recreation, education is a dangerous one.

PINK   36. Men have more inherent ability to think logically than do women.

WHITE   37. Men have the advantage in our society because they have power and status.

GREEN   38. A woman can best achieve full self-development by getting the best education and training possible.

PINK   39. Most women do not want to be independent,
but want a man to take care of them.

YELLOW   40. Man's inherent strengths are different from
woman's, and these strengths complement
each other.

YELLOW   41. Women are naturally more expressive emotionally than men, and any moves toward
"liberation" should enhance this quality.

WHITE   42. Child care should be provided by the state
for all who want it.

PINK   43. Generally speaking, men do not have the emotional make-up to stay home and assume the
domestic role.

WHITE   44. Most men are afraid of strong and competent
women.

WHITE   45. Men and women can best overcome discrimination through the revolutionary overthrow
of the present system.

PINK   46. Women have the advantage in our society
because they have protection, leisure, and
freedom from the pressure to achieve.

PINK   47.   A man can best achieve full self-development by being a good husband and provider.

YELLOW 48.   Women can best overcome discrimination by working individually to prove their abilities.

GREEN   49.   Men treat women as toys.

WHITE   50.   Men and women have the same biological (genetic) range of emotional and intellectual capacities. The differences present in our society are all learned.

WHITE   51.   Women can best overcome discrimination by working in exclusively female groups.

GREEN   52.   Men neglect issues of health and welfare, and therefore women are appropriate political leaders for our country.

WHITE   53.   Almost all men are sexists—either consciously or unconsciously.

YELLOW 54.   Women are really the "stronger sex"—they provide emotional support for the man so he can achieve. "Behind every great man there is a woman."

PINK   55.   The husband should have the final decision on important matters.

YELLOW 56.   A woman can best achieve full self-development by taking a job that utilizes the unique skills and qualities that she has.

Scoring Sheet

ATTITUDES: Old Masculinist ("biology is destiny")

New Masculinist ("vive la difference, but down with discrimination")

Old Feminist ("anything men can do, women can do better")

New Feminist ("sex-linked roles are obsolete")

SCORING YOUR CHOICES: Give each slip the "weight" of the pile into which you sorted it. If a slip is in pile #7, give it 7 in the scorebox to the right of the slip color; if a slip is in pile #3, write down 3 in the scorebox. Add up the points in each scorebox and enter the total in the appropriate column. A high score represents an identification with that attitude.

ATTITUDE	SLIP COLOR	SCOREBOX	TOTAL
Old masculinist	pink		
New masculinist	yellow		
Old feminist	green		
New feminist	white		

※   ※   ※

SUBJECT: *Completion of "I AM . . ." Sentences*

MATERIALS NEEDED:

Ten slips of paper for each person.
Pencil for each person.

TIME REQUIRED: 20-30 minutes.

OBJECTIVES:

To increase personal awareness of how individuals see themselves, their roles, their personal characteristics.

To clarify what significance different personality characteristics or roles have for each person.

To receive further clarification and feedback through sharing with others in the group.

RATIONALE:

While this exercise is not an exploration of male-female roles, it is helpful in the value approach to sexuality for persons to describe themselves and to discover whether or not they see their identity primarily in terms of a role (student, parent, etc.) or as individuals with particular skills, interests, feelings.

Through the process of rank ordering (see step 3 of the PROCEDURE) the "I AM . . ." slips, persons often may gain new insights about their own needs and about the positive and negative functions their behavior characteristics (roles) serve for them.

PROCEDURE:

1. Form into trios.

2. Leader distributes slips of paper, ten to each person, then says:

   "On each of these slips, tell something about your-self by completing the sentence "I AM . . ." Trust the first things that come into your head about who you are and put them down."

3. When students have completed ten sentences, give the following directions:

   "You now have ten slips of paper which describe you. Some you probably regard as more important than others. Stack the slips in order of importance to you, with the most important on top."

4. After this is done, continue:

   "Look at the way you have arranged the slips. Look for any patterns which may exist among those slips on the top and those on the bottom. Ask yourself: 'Are there any I'd like to throw away? What do I gain or lose by retaining this characteristic'?"

5. Allow a few minutes for each person to do this. Then say:

   "Now share with the other two people in your trio what you have written on your slips, and your feelings and reactions about them. Partners may ask clarifying questions, but should be nonjudgmental."

6. NOTE TO LEADER: Some individuals may list roles (teacher, mother, husband, etc.) to characterize themselves, while others may list personal aspects (creative, critical, dependent, etc.). It is useful to call this to people's attention, and suggest that they think about the different implications of the two approaches.

OTHER SUGGESTIONS
FOR EXPLORING SEX ROLES IN OUR SOCIETY

1. *Sex Roles in Popular Songs*

Tape some of the popular songs of the day, and some old songs. Have participants form in small groups and give them the task of listening to a group of old songs and listing the sexual stereotypes which distinguish the male and female roles. Then do the same for the modern songs. Compare the two lists for differences and similarities.

This exercise could be done in mixed-sex groups or same-sex groups. If it is done in same-sex caucuses, it would be instructive to have a male group join with a female group and compare lists. Another possibility is to post lists—male on one wall and female on the other—and then discuss the differences in perceptions.

2. *Collage of Sex Stereotypes*

Bring many magazines to the meeting—family, men's,

women's, and children's. Form small same-sex groups,
and give each group some magazines. Have the men
make a collage of the American woman, using pictures
from the magazines, and ask them to list the stereotypes
most commonly found. Have the women do a similar
collage and list for the men.

Then, depending on the size of the class: post the
collages and have the women respond to the men's work;
then have the men respond to the women's; *or*, if the class
is too large, have each women's group join with a men's
group and discuss the other's collage and list.

3. *Role Reversal Greetings*

Form into several same-sex groupings. Each woman's
group join a men's group. Flip a coin to see who will go
first. As the group which goes first proceeds with the exercise, the opposite-sex group watches without talking. The
directions are:

   a. "Greet each person in your group in the manner you
      feel would be characteristic of the *opposite sex*. You
      may touch or not, as you wish, but do not speak.

   b. "When you have greeted each person in your group,
      then begin greeting again, only this time in the man-
      ner you feel is characteristic of *your own sex.*

   c. "Now, talk with the members of your group about the
      experience. How did you feel in each situation? What
      male or female stereotypes did you observe?

   d. "After you have made all the observations you care to,

invite comment from members of the opposite-sex caucus which watched. How did they perceive what you did?"

Repeat the whole procedure, with the observer group now doing the greeting.

VALUES CLARIFICATION

SUBJECT: *Patterns of Value Choices*

MATERIALS NEEDED:

None—just a large room so several small groups can converse simultaneously.

TIME REQUIRED: Indefinite.

OBJECTIVES:

To choose what's most important and least important from a field of options.

To share the reasoning behind your choices of values with others who may not subscribe to your values.

To experience personal interaction in several small groups.

RATIONALE:

In order to choose one alternative and reject others, the students have to examine their feelings and their values. This process helps the individuals clarify what is really important to them.

Having to justify choice forces a person to look carefully at the decision and evaluate it clearly.

This exercise serves as a good ice-breaker for a large group and/or a new group. It provides an opportunity to meet many individuals and to discuss important and personal issues at the outset.

PROCEDURE:

1. Introduce the exercise to the entire class:

    "We are going to do an exercise called values clarification, and in the process we will get together briefly with several different groups of people.
    "I will read a set of three statements. Each of you is to choose which of the three is the most important in your life, and which is least important. Then you will break off into groups and discuss the assumptions that underlie your choice."

2. It is important that individuals do not take a great deal of time to make their decisions, but trust their initial response. After discussing their choices with the group, they may discover that they would have chosen differently if they had taken into account this factor or that, or they may find they can trust their spontaneous reactions to bear up under scrutiny.

3. Read the first set of statements:

    "Which of the following three do you consider the most important to you, and which is the least important?

Trust your initial response and stay with it. There is no right or wrong answer.

"For me, it is most important that a sexual experience:

    a. "Be fun and pleasurable.

    b. "Increase the possibility of honesty and openness.

    c. "Enhance self-respect."

4. Read the statements through a second time. Then direct the participants to break up into groups.

    There are several options for doing this. Take the first set of statements as an example, and use the following shorthand to designate the choices:

    (1) Fun

    (2) Honest

    (3) Self-respect

    A, B, C, D, E, etc. to designate areas of the room

    I. After the leader reads the statements in set (1), people may be directed to group for discussion in the following ways:

    A. All who put (1) as most important.
    B. All who put (2) as most important.
    C. All who put (3) as most important.

or

II.   A, B, C as above, then:
Those at A who put (2) as least important go to D.
Those at A who put (3) as least important go to E.

Those at B who put (1) as least important go to F.
Those at B who put (3) as least important go to G.

Those at C who put (1) as least important go to H.
Those at C who put (2) as least important go to I.

or

III.   A.   A random one-fifth of the group.
B.   A random one-fifth of the group.
C.   A random one-fifth of the group.
D.   A random one-fifth of the group.
E.   A random one-fifth of the group.

If method II is used after the reading of each set, it will provide for a variety of discussion partners (unless the group is homogeneous on every issue).

5.   When all participants have formed into groups, say:

"Ask questions to explore what assumptions underlie the choices of those in your group. You may discover that these assumptions are very different, even for the same choices. Ask yourself, 'What made me choose this statement rather than one of the others? What does that tell me about myself?'

"Avoid being judgmental toward those who have different reasons for their choices than you do; instead, try to understand what these people are trying to communicate."

Give five to ten minutes for sharing each time you present a set of statements.

6.   Other sets of statements:

II.   Of the following three activities, the most important and the least important to me is:
    a.   To spend an evening with a close friend.
    b.   To spend a beautiful day outdoors.
    c.   To have a good orgasm.

III.   If I am feeling the need for release of sexual tension, I would rather:
    a.   Masturbate.
    b.   Screw.
    c.   Engage in vigorous physical activity.

IV.   In a sexual relationship, I would prefer that:
    a.   Sex be more meaningful to me than to the other person.
    b.   Sex be more meaningful to the other person than to me.
    c.   Sex be meaningful to neither one of us.

V.   The worst thing that I could find out about my boyfriend or girlfriend, husband or wife is that my mate:
    a.   Has syphilis.
    b.   Is sterile.
    c.   Is promiscuous.

7.   If you want to bring diversity to the surface and promote discussion between persons with different values, then you can put together the groups in a different way. Depending upon the size of the class, you can either have

participants stay in their last group and reflect and share, or come back together into a full class to look at such questions as:

Did any of you find a pattern in your responses?
Did some particular values surface again and again?
What was this experience like for you?
What made it easy or hard to share your feelings—subject matter, persons you were with, ways people interacted, etc....?

☙   ☙   ☙

SUBJECT: *Card Drawing and Sexual Attitudes*

MATERIALS NEEDED:

Overhead projector or a chart.
For each small group, one envelope containing set of eight cards, with one of the eight topics to be discussed written on each card. Possible topics are:

Virginity	*Oral-genital sex*
Intercourse	*Masturbation*
Sterilization	*Group sex*
Homosexuality	*Extramarital relations*
Abortion	

Nudity—with acquaintances, with family, with opposite sex, with same sex, with close friends.
Physical closeness and touching—with casual acquaintances, with close friends, with same sex, with opposite sex, with boy (girl) friend.

TIME REQUIRED: Indefinite (minimum one hour).

OBJECTIVES:

To identify and express present attitudes and feelings about a variety of sexual matters.

To identify and to share the incongruencies which often exist between what we think and what we feel.

To practice active listening and honest self-disclosure.

To become aware of the group's diversity of viewpoints related to sexual matters.

RATIONALE:

In our culture, individuals often need a structure which gives them permission to talk about sexual concerns. Through this focused sharing, individuals are able to clarify what they feel and believe, and to identify when there is a discrepancy between head and gut.

Group members will be more trusting and more willing to discuss personal feelings and attitudes if: (1) they feel free to say that they don't want to talk about a given subject; and (2) if they feel they are being listened to in a nonjudgmental way. Special attention should be given in the introduction and directions to these two prerequisites for success.

PROCEDURE:

1.   Form into groups of six.

2.   Leader introduces exercise:

"For most people talking about sexual attitudes in a group like this is a relatively new experience. But it is a fruitful experience, because often you may discover that others share the feelings and attitudes that you may have felt were unique to you and that you may therefore have been reluctant to talk about.

"Also, clarifying our attitudes and beliefs by talking them over with people makes us more conscious of what we feel. Therefore, our feelings are more subject to our rational powers of choice, rather than we being subject to or driven by our feelings.

"We are not trying to *change* anybody's attitude or value; we are trying to bring to your consciousness what your attitudes and values are. Liberality is not necessarily the "good" position, nor is conservatism (or traditional values) necessarily the "bad" one. The important thing is what *you* affirm and espouse.

"The intention of this exercise is to make it possible for people to express whatever value they hold—which means that in your groups, don't argue, just try to listen and respond nonjudgmentally. Let the person expressing himself/herself know you understand—not just by saying "I understand," but by relaying back the essence of what was said, as you heard it. Practice trying to accept *whatever* a person says. But then, take the risk of saying what *you* believe, even if you think your feelings are different from those of everyone else in the group.

"So, then, today we are going to explore some of our sexual attitudes regarding the subjects here on the overhead [chart]."

3.   Project transparency, or display chart, with the eight

areas listed. It is important to post the areas of discussion so that participants are not taken unawares, and thus threatened, by the topics. Say:

"We will be talking about these areas, not only in regard to ourselves, but also how we feel about masturbation, for instance, for our mates or friends. We will also be checking on ourselves to see whether our head and gut are together (in my head, I think masturbation is normal and healthy; in my gut, I still feel some uneasiness and guilt about it).

"Now, one person in each group take the eight cards out of the envelope and place them face down in the center of your group. Another person is then to draw first. The material on the cards is the same as what is posted here (indicate chart or overhead). If you are unwilling to talk about your attitudes on the topic you draw, put that card back and draw another.

"Let me review the procedure briefly: After you have drawn the card and read the topic aloud, you are the first to respond, saying: how you feel in regard to talking about this topic; how you feel about this topic for yourself, for others, in general, and for persons close to you; whether your head and gut are together. When you are finished, another person in the group will draw a card and speak first. Each individual will take a turn at drawing."

4. NOTE TO LEADER: It is important to guard against the tendency of a group to focus exclusively on the person who draws the card—asking questions, responding, drawing that person out—in other words, keeping that one individual on the hot seat. This prevents a *total group* sharing. It is easier and less risky to keep the focus on

another person, rather than revealing one's own attitudes and values.

❃   ❃   ❃

SUBJECT: *Sexual Behavior Continuum*

MATERIALS NEEDED:

Two sexual-values continuums (see pages 107-111 for models).
A large sheet of paper to tabulate group results.
Felt-tip pen or crayon.
For Alternative Procedure: Masking tape.
Tagboard signs (3).

TIME REQUIRED: 15-45 minutes.

OBJECTIVES:

To provide a mechanism which forces students to "declare themselves" on specified sexual issues.

To generate a group profile with regard to attitudes on specified sexual issues.

To facilitate comparison of students' attitudes.

RATIONALE:

One necessary ingredient for group building is a flow of information among the group members, so that increasingly they know where each member stands on a variety of issues.

It is sometimes interesting and useful to portray in graph or continuum form the attitude profile of a particular group. This serves the function of revealing commonalities and illuminating differences.

PROCEDURE: Alternative I

1.   Form groups of six. Hand out two values continuums—one on sexual behavior, the other on sexual practices and the law. Review the directions with the students, then allow about 10 minutes for them to complete the continuums.

2.   To get a picture of the diversity and/or similarity within a group, instruct the participants to tabulate their results in a large continuum on one sheet of newsprint.

3.   Discuss in small groups any observations or concerns people have.

PROCEDURE: Alternative II

1.   Make the continuum line on the floor with masking tape. Lay cardboard signs along the line to demarcate the positions.

2.   Introduce the exercise:

"You see here on the floor a large continuum. I am going to call out a sexual behavior. Will each of you get

up and move to the position on the continuum which represents your viewpoint about that behavior."

3. Call off the first item on the list. After everyone has taken
    a position, say:

    "Now look about you at the people who agree with
    you and those who disagree with you. Talk for a few
    moments with those nearest you about how you feel
    being where you are and why. Then return to your
    places."

4. Continue with each item, varying the directions now and
    then by asking people to move toward someone who is
    standing at an opposite position from themselves, and to
    talk with that person about the issues.

5. At the conclusion of the exercise, gather in small groups
    to talk about any observations growing out of the activity.

Sexual Practices and the Law

Where would you place the following on the continuum below? Write the number at the appropriate place.

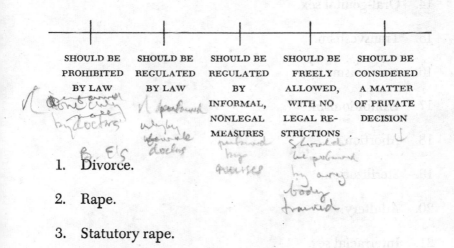

| SHOULD BE PROHIBITED BY LAW | SHOULD BE REGULATED BY LAW | SHOULD BE REGULATED BY INFORMAL, NONLEGAL MEASURES | SHOULD BE FREELY ALLOWED, WITH NO LEGAL RESTRICTIONS | SHOULD BE CONSIDERED A MATTER OF PRIVATE DECISION |

1. Divorce.

2. Rape.

3. Statutory rape.

4. Child molestation.

5. Publication of pornographic material.

6. Display of pornographic material.

7. Dissemination of contraceptive information.

8. Distribution of contraceptive devices.

9. Display of contraceptive devices.

10. Marital sexual behavior.

11. Nonmarital cohabitation.

12. Prostitution.

13. Soliciting.

14. Oral-genital sex.

15. Transvestism.

16. Voyeurism.

17. Exhibitionism.

18. Abortion.

19. Sterilization.

20. Adultery.

21. Interracial sex.

22. Masturbation.

23. Incest.

24. Polygamy.

25. Nuisance "sexual" phone calls and letters.

26. Homosexual cohabitation.

27. Homosexual soliciting.

28. Sex education.

29. Nudity.

※   ※   ※

Sexual Behavior

Read each item and reflect individually on how you feel about that behavior *right now*. Then identify where that behavior would fit on your continuum line, and write the number for that behavior at that point on the line.

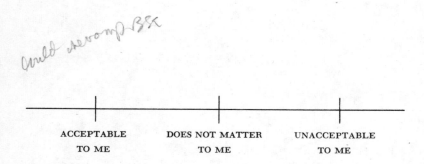

1. Homosexuality for myself as a life style.

2. Homosexuality for others as a life style.

3. Technical virginity—"everything but."

4. Virginity before marriage.

5. Double standard of sexual behavior for men and women.

6. Egalitarian masculine-feminine roles.

7. Sex without love.

8. Sex with love.

9. Masturbation.

10. Marriage.

11. Tenderness as a condition for sex.

12. Women's liberation.

13. Men's liberation.

14. Abortion for myself or partner.

15. Petting to orgasm.

16. Promiscuity.

17. Interracial sex.

18. Extramarital sex.

19. Group sex.

20. Sexual initiative always taken by me.

21. Sexual initiative always taken by partner.

22. Bisexuality for myself as a life style.

23. Bisexuality for others as a life style.

24. Oral-genital sex.

※   ※   ※

SUBJECT: *Consensus Exercise*

MATERIALS NEEDED:

Paper and pencil for each person.
Overhead projector with transparency, or chart, listing cast
of characters.

TIME REQUIRED: 60-90 minutes.

OBJECTIVES:

To identify, verbalize, and clarify personal value positions.

To increase awareness of the assumptions underlying our
judgements and values.

To become aware of dogmatism and ambivalence in self and
others.

RATIONALE:

Focusing on the behavior of fictional characters rather than on
oneself or one's acquaintances is sometimes a useful and nonthreatening way of examining one's own values.

Most of us are unaware of many of the assumptions on which
we operate, and hence are unclear about how we reach certain
decisions. Through the process of trying to reach group consensus, underlying assumptions are surfaced.

In the consensus process, individual behavior is usually consistent with behavior in similar situations in "the real world." This exercise illuminates typical response patterns.

PROCEDURE:

1.   Form groups of six.

2.   Place on overhead or write on chart the cast of persons in the story, in order of their appearance:

> DAVID—Beth's fiancé
>
> BETH—David's fiancée
>
> CARL—Beth's classmate
>
> ANN—Beth's close friend
>
> EDWARD—Beth's new acquaintance

Leave this list visible, so participants can see it throughout the exercise.

3.   Leader introduces the exercise:

"Today I am going to tell you a story about the people whose names are written here on the overhead—David, Beth, Carl, Ann, and Edward.

"David and Beth are engaged to be married. David is away in the service, stationed in Alaska. Beth is still in school, and shares a class with Carl. She and Carl become friends. They sleep together. Beth decides she doesn't feel right about having intercourse with Carl and tells him they'll have to stop. They do.

"Some time passes. Carl tells Beth he is driving to Alaska. Beth asks Carl to take her along, so she can see David. Carl says, 'Okay, if you'll go to bed with me.'

"Beth is uncertain what to do. She talks to Ann about it. She and Ann are close friends. Ann says, 'Do what you think is best.' Beth decides to go to bed with Carl.

"Meanwhile, David has been dating, on a casual basis, a nurse stationed near him in Alaska. When Beth gets to Alaska, she feels obliged to tell David about her relationship with Carl. David breaks off the engagement, says he can't trust Beth.

"Beth returns home. She meets Edward. She is upset and tells him all. Edward asks her to live with him.

"The end."

4. Instruct each person to take out a piece of paper and a pencil, and without any discussion, to rank the five people in the story, number 1 being the one he/she likes best, and number 5 being the one he/she likes least.

5. When the ranking is complete, have the groups split into two trios. (If the group continues to consist of six people, there is not enough time for everyone to have "air time," and the process of trying to reach consensus is much more complicated and frustrating.)

6. When all the groups have divided into trios, give the following directions:

"In your trios, compare your rankings of the characters. Give reasons for your choices, and try to reach a consensus, so that all three lists will agree. You have 10 minutes to reach consensus."

7. Instruct trios to reform into groups of six, to share their rankings and discuss where they agreed and disagreed, and why.

8. Some of the issues which may emerge both in the consensus of three, and in the sharing of six, are:

   a. The role of honesty in a relationship.

   b. The relationship between emotional commitment and sexual intercourse.

   c. Exploitation in a personal relationship.

   d. When intercourse is appropriate.

   e. The role of a friend.

   f. The double standard.

   g. The meaning of engagement.

                    ☼   ☼   ☼

SUBJECT: *Self-Picture—Where I Am*

                    Where I'd Like to Be

MATERIALS NEEDED:

   Three large sheets of newsprint per person.
   Crayons or paints.

TIME REQUIRED: 75-120 minutes.

OBJECTIVES:

To express graphically how one sees oneself sexually.

To provide a means by which personal feelings about sexuality may be shared within a small group.

To clarify the relationship of past experience, present situation, and desired future situation.

RATIONALE:

It is sometimes productive to use methods other than verbal exchange for helping people reflect on the meanings they attach to their own sexuality. Although many participants will protest that they are not "artists," it is revealing how accurately the colors, forms, and symbols used by "non-artists" do communicate what they want to express. People often find themselves "painted by the picture," and saying, "I just put this color or that shape down. When I was drawing it, I didn't really have a reason—but now I can see that it means _____ to me."

The visual form makes a more memorable sharing medium—people often can remember a person's drawing many months after they have forgotten the person's words.

PROCEDURE:

1. Give the following directions:

         "After each of you has completed an individual period of reflection and drawing, you will be communicating in very small groups (three or four persons).

"Number the three sheets of newsprint I have provided. Now take sheet #1, and draw "Where You Are *Now*, Sexually." Portray whatever appears to you as a characteristic of your sexuality at the present. This is not an art competition, so use stick figures, abstractions, or whatever you find best expresses the gist of your own situation."

2. After almost everyone has completed drawing #1, announce:

"Those of you who have finished picture #1, now take #2 and draw "Where You Would Like to Be Sexually." (Put these directions on board or chart so individuals who finish #1 later can continue to #2 without interruption.)

3. After almost everyone has completed drawing #2, announce:

"On the last sheet, portray 'What Would Have to Happen, to Move from Where I Am to Where I Would Like to Be.'"

4. When students have finished their drawings, say:

"Find two or three other people who have also finished, and quietly move to a place where you can share your drawings without disturbing people who are still working."

※   ※   ※

SUBJECT: *What I Value in a Sexual Relationship*

MATERIALS NEEDED:

Sheet of paper and a pencil or pen for each person.

TIME REQUIRED: 20-40 minutes.

OBJECTIVES:

To identify what each person values in a sexual relationship.

To give students practice in sorting out priorities, and in publicly affirming and explaining what is most important to them in a sexual relationship.

RATIONALE:

The task of writing down what one values in a sexual relationship requires a sorting and decision-making process.

This exercise provides an opportunity for individuals to examine and learn about diverse value orientations.

PROCEDURE: Alternative I

1.   Instruct participants to form groups of five or six.

2.   Then say:

"Mark off your sheet of paper into eight boxes. In each box write one thing which you value in a sexual relationship."

3. After a few minutes have passed, instruct the students to tear apart the eight boxes so that each thing they value is on a separate slip of paper.

    "Now that you each have eight slips of paper, rank order these slips, putting on top the one which is most important to you, and on bottom the one which is least important to you."

4. Allow a few minutes for individuals to complete this process. Then give these instructions:

    "Now, one person in each group volunteer to go first and share your rank ordering with the group. Listeners should ask questions about whatever will help them understand what the sharer means and how he/she feels. Try to do this in a nonjudgmental way. Point out where you disagree with the sharer and tell your reasons for disagreeing. Be sure everyone has a chance to disclose his/her rank-order in this group discussion."

5. It is helpful to warn the group members a few minutes before it is time to terminate the exercise that their time is almost over. Also, it is often instructive to invite the participants to get together as a total class and share what they learned from this exercise.

PROCEDURE: Alternative II

Since the use of eight slips generates a great deal of material to choose a partner, with whom he/she will share his/her list in any way the two of them find helpful. With only two persons, each can speak at more length than in a group of five or six or in a total-class sharing.

OTHER SUGGESTIONS FOR CLARIFYING VALUES IN SEXUALITY

Exercise 1.

List what you feel are the three most important changes you would like to see in attitudes toward sexuality among:

    a. Society

    b. Parents

    c. Peers

    d. Males

    e. Females

Choose one or more of these categories for discussion.

Exercise 2.

Draw a line down the center of a piece of paper. On one side, list:

    What I'd like most *now* in a relationship that includes sexual expression.

On the other side, list:

    What I'd like *10 years from now* in a relationship that includes sexual expression.

Compare and discuss lists. Defend choices. Help others clarify their choices.

Exercise 3.

Each person has a 3 x 5 card. On one side, list:
   What I value most about my own sexuality.

On the other side, list:
   What others value most about my sexuality.

In small groups, note and discuss discrepancies in the two lists. Help one another clarify what effect those differences have on the individual.

Explore ways of dealing with those differences.

See if there are some common elements in the lists of the students.

Exercise 4.

Each person has a 3 x 5 card. On one side, list:
   Two words related to my sexuality which I'd *most* like to have used in reference to me.

On the other side, list:
   Two words related to my sexuality which I'd *least* like to have used in reference to me.

Share and discuss in small groups.

DIMENSIONS IN RELATIONSHIPS

Introduction to the Use
of Nonverbal Techniques

THE USE OF NONVERBAL TECHNIQUES, followed by a reflection and sharing period, provides the participants with an opportunity to discover how much is communicated without words in all our interactions with others. This can be a powerful tool for providing insight into how one typically interacts with another person, how one feels about one's style of interaction, and whether or not this differs according to sex.

In these exercises the student sees how stereotypical sex roles relate to how people interact. Nonverbal exercises also aid in exploring the dimensions of intimacy and control within a relationship.

Most frequently, the chief learning value of a nonverbal exercise comes in the discussion which follows the nonverbal part of the procedure. In this discussion the students reflect on and verbalize how they felt about what they and their partner(s) did in the nonverbal segment. This process adds clarity and cognition to what otherwise might remain vague feelings.

Those engaged in an intimate relationship often assume that their partner knows what he/she wants and likes. This assumption causes much hurt and pain in many relationships. Unless they are endowed with E.S.P., individuals in a relationship must break down this inhibition and communicate intimate feelings to each other. Hopefully, the nonverbal experiences which follow will help make this kind of communication a natural and ongoing part of a relationship.

Exercises Which Explore Intimacy:

> Table Top Scramble (see Group-Building Activities)
>
> Hand Exploration
>
> Physical Closeness and Nonverbal Mill
>
> Foot Massage
>
> Role-Reversal Greeting (see Sex Roles)

Exercises Which Explore Control, Initiation, and Kinds of Power:

> Hand Exploration
>
> Fist Opening
>
> Mirroring

SUBJECT: *Hand Exploration*

MATERIALS NEEDED: None.

TIME REQUIRED: 15 minutes.

OBJECTIVES:

To communicate feelings nonverbally.

To increase self-awareness of how one expresses different feelings and how one feels about one's own style of expression.

To experience feelings in interaction with another person, to share those feelings verbally, and to discover how the other person felt about the same experience.

RATIONALE:

The prospect of communicating nonverbally frequently arouses resistance and anxiety in individuals who have not experienced this type of activity before. Because our society does not view hand contact as intimate, using the hands to explore feelings is a nonthreatening way to introduce issues related to intimate communication.

Through the experience of expressing anger, affection, strength, playfullness, etc., with one's hands, without being able to verbalize, participants often become aware, in a new way, of which emotions engender discomfort, awkwardness, or pleasure.

The verbal sharing with one's partner of what each person experienced builds trust. It also increases the possibility that such sharing will take place in other relationships.

PROCEDURE:

1. Give the following instructions:

    "Find a partner, preferably someone you do not know very well, and sit down, facing each other."

2. When everyone has a partner, continue the instructions:

    "You and your partner are going to do a nonverbal hand exploration. I will give directions from the center. Close your eyes, and without talking, take your partner's hand. Get to know each other's hand, feel the texture, the shape; explore the fingers."

3. Allow a few minutes between each step. Tell them to:

    a. "Express impatience with your partner; fight with each other.

    b. "Now make up; be affectionate, caring to each other.

    c. "Communicate your strength to your partner; test your power and strength with each other.

    d. "Play with each other; what ways can you discover to be playful with your partner's hand?

    e. "Now express hesitancy, questioning to your

partner; communicate that you are uncertain about this relationship.

f.   "Move from hesitancy to detachment; pull back, put up a wall—in some way detach yourself as a human being while still maintaining touch.

g.   "Now come back and simply *be there* for your partner.

"When you feel ready, separate and put your hand in your lap. Then share with your partner how you felt during this exercise. What parts of the exercise did you find most comfortable? most uncomfortable?"

5.   After the partners have had time to discuss and share their feelings (about three to five minutes), it is often helpful to learn how others experienced the exercise by having a total class discussion. The questions to focus on might be the following:

What did you learn about yourself in this exercise? What implications does what you learned have for you as a man or a woman?

�€   ☀   ☀

SUBJECT: *Physical Closeness and Nonverbal Mill*

MATERIALS NEEDED:

Checklist for each individual (see page 130 for model).

TIME REQUIRED: 15-20 minutes.

OBJECTIVES:

To provide a "laboratory" (contrived) experience of physical interaction and eye contact as the basis for identifying and discussing attitudes about intimacy.

To identify customary personal responses to situations of physical closeness.

RATIONALE:

One of the issues in sexual interaction (and any personal interaction, for that matter) is the individual's tolerance for various degrees of closeness. This exercise is designed to be a "low-threat" way of helping individuals identify their customary style of reacting to physical closeness and eye contact.

Because this is a contrived situation rather than a spontaneous one, people's reactions will not exactly duplicate their ordinary responses. But if people will keep touch with their feelings toward various encounters, this exercise will prove productive.

PROCEDURE:

1. Instruct class to move to an open place in the room where they can mill around freely.

    "We are going to engage in an experiment regarding your reactions to physical closeness. This will be most useful to you if you can recognize your reactions to various encounters relating to the dimension of closeness.

"This is a contrived situation, so your responses here will not represent exactly the responses you might have with a group of friends. But if you focus attention on your own reactions, you will learn something about the way you act to close physical encounters with those of the same sex and with those of the opposite sex.

"From now on, please remain silent, since you can learn most from this exercise when there is no speaking.

"Here are the directions: When I signal you to begin, you are to mill around in your group, encountering each person in the group individually, and moving a little closer to him/her than you normally would. Look in the person's eyes. Nonverbally, decide when to move on.

"This is not a feedback exercise—you are not necessarily expressing how you feel about the people in your group. You are simply learning about your own feelings toward physical encounter. You may touch or not, depending on each of you, but this is not primarily a touching exercise—it is a clarification of your responses to intimacy and closeness.

"Return to your places when you have encountered everyone in the manner I have just explained."

2. When everyone is seated, give each student a checklist which looks like the one on page 130.

3. Then say:

"This is a checklist to help you reflect on how you felt during the nonverbal mill. After you have filled it out, look at it carefully to see what patterns of reaction seem to emerge, and whether these are characteristic behaviors for you in other situations. The checklist is for your own use. You are under no obligation to share what you put down, unless you wish to do so."

4. Allow a few minutes for the students to fill out the check-list. When most seem finished, invite them to break off into informal small groups and share any feelings or reactions to the exercise that they wish to share.

Physical Closeness and Nonverbal Mill

PERSONAL CHECKLIST
(not to be shared unless you want to)

In the milling activity, I was:

COMFORTABLE WITH		UNCOMFORTABLE WITH
_____	The physical closeness	_____
_____	The eye contact	_____
_____	Touching	_____
_____	People of same sex	_____
_____	People of opposite sex	_____
_____	The nonverbal communication	_____
_____	My initiating	_____
_____	Having the other person initiate	_____
_____	Other (specify)	_____

When I felt uncomfortable, I

_____	Moved away
_____	Backed off
_____	Looked away
_____	Laughed or grinned
_____	Looked down
_____	Felt angry
_____	Other
_____	These responses are fairly typical of my responses in similar situations.
_____	These responses are not typical of me.

⚜   ⚜   ⚜

SUBJECT: *Foot Massage*

MATERIALS NEEDED: None.

TIME REQUIRED: 10-30 minutes.

OBJECTIVES:

To express physical caring to another person.

To increase sensory awareness, and to gain acceptance of a part of the body we seldom appreciate.

To practice telling a partner what is pleasurable to you and what is not.

RATIONALE:

See Introduction to The Use of Nonverbal Techniques.

PROCEDURE:

1.   Direct students to find a partner, without talking, preferably someone they haven't paired with before, or don't know well. After ascertaining that everyone has a partner, say:

    "We are going to do a foot massage. Decide who shall be the first to give and the first to receive. Get in a comfortable position, and take off your shoes and socks."

2.   It may be helpful to say something to acknowledge and

relieve the anxiety or embarrassment some people might have about their feet being dirty.

3.   Be sure to allow a few minutes between each step.

    a.   "Take one foot in your hands. Both partners close their eyes. Giver, feel the weight of that foot. Receiver, feel the hands on your foot, holding it.

    b.   "Press firmly against the foot with your hands.

    c.   "Giver, open your eyes and begin slapping the foot. Starting at the heel, slap the foot firmly, being sure to cover the entire foot.

    d.   "Now, slapping lightly, slap the entire foot again. Don't forget the toes.

    e.   "Massage the foot, at first firmly and then more gently.

    f.   "Care for that foot in whatever way you wish. When you feel ready to stop, gently place the foot on the floor.

    g.   "Receiver, when you feel ready, open your eyes. Both giver and receiver, share with your partner what the experiment was like."

4.   Allow a few minutes for sharing, then interrupt:

    "Many of us find it difficult to tell our partner what feels good and what doesn't. We often think our partner is supposed to just *know;* to read our minds somehow.

Unfortunately, it doesn't often work that way.

"Receiver, before your partner massages your other foot, tell him or her what you particularly liked, what you want more of; if there was something you didn't like, now is the time to say so."

5. Allow a brief time for this conversation to take place, then continue:

    "Giver, take the other foot of your partner. Hold it firmly in both hands. Look at that foot, be aware of its shape, its skin texture, its uniqueness.

    "Now care for that foot in whatever way you wish, keeping in mind what your partner just told you."

6. After about three minutes (or longer, if time permits), tell the givers to complete the massage and to place the foot gently on the floor.

7. Instruct students to change places with their partners.

8. Repeat steps 3 through 6.

9. At this point, you may choose to have a total class sharing. Some possible questions for initiating the sharing process:

    How do you feel about yourself and your partner after doing this exercise?

    What did you learn about yourself?

    How did those of you who were with members of the same sex feel?

Was it hard to tell your partner what you liked?

What implications do you see for sexual interaction from this exercise?

※   ※   ※

SUBJECT: *Fist Opening*

MATERIALS NEEDED:

Overhead projector and transparency or chart listing questions (optional).

TIME REQUIRED: 10-20 minutes.

OBJECTIVE:

To explore personal styles of persuading and responding, and issues of control and perseverance.

RATIONALE:

See Introduction to The Use of Nonverbal Techniques.

PROCEDURE:

1. It is most fruitful to do this exercise twice: if possible, with a member of the same sex, and then with a member of the opposite sex. But even if the class makeup does not

permit this, it is advisable for each student to do the exercise with two different partners. Doing this exercise twice gives each person an opportunity to try a new behavior. It also increases awareness of the diversity of styles of behavior, as well as an individual's own responses to different behaviors.

2. Give the following directions:

"Without talking, choose a partner and stand facing one another. This is a fist-opening exercise. One person in each pair make a tight fist, holding your arm out toward your partner. The task is to get your partner's fist open. Do this without talking. When you have succeeded in opening your partner's fist, change places. When both of you have opened the other's fist, sit down."

3. Allow about five minutes for the partners to share their perceptions about the exercise.

4. Give next set of directions:

"Now find a new partner (of the opposite sex, if possible). Nonverbally, decide who will be first to make a fist. Repeat the exercise. You might want to try a new behavior this time and see how that feels, or you may want to do it the same way and see how a different partner responds to the same behavior. Try to keep in touch with what you're feeling as you do this."

5. When the pairs have finished, the leader may place on the overhead and/or read the following questions for reflection and sharing between the members of pairs.

How do you feel about what just happened between you?

What did opening or not opening the fist mean to you?

What made you open your fist?

How do you feel about: (1) power; (2) seduction; (3) playfulness as a way of getting someone to do something?

Did the sex of your partner make a difference? How?

6. It may be helpful to have the total class share their responses to such questions as:

What did you learn about yourself in doing this exercise?

How did the sex of your partner affect your behavior feelings?

※   ※   ※

SUBJECT: *Mirroring*

MATERIALS NEEDED:

Chart or overhead projector with transparency (optional).

TIME REQUIRED: 5-10 minutes.

OBJECTIVES:

To increase awareness of one's personal style of relating to another person.

To explore issues of control and initiation-response.

RATIONALE:

See Introduction to The Use of Nonverbal Techniques.

PROCEDURE:

1.   Give the following directions:

"Without talking, find a partner, someone you haven't been with before or don't know well. Then find a space in the room where you can stretch in all directions without touching anyone."

2.   After everyone has a partner, say:

"You and your partner are going to do a nonverbal exercise called mirroring. You are to mirror what your partner does. Stand facing each other, and place the palms of your hands on your partner's hands. Look into each other's eyes. Now, keeping your hands in the same position, separate them from your partner's slightly. You should not be touching each other.

"Explore the space around you, one person mirroring the movements of the other."

3. Allow a few minutes between each step.

    a. "Express who you are with movements.

    b. "Now slow down, move in slow motion.

    c. "Express how you are feeling right now.

    d. "Close, tell your partner good-bye.

    e. "When you have finished, sit down with your partner and share how you feel about what you just did together."

4. The leader may wish to guide discussion. The following questions could be read and/or placed on a chart or overhead projector.

    How did the two of you resolve the leadership issue?

    Is this consistent with your behavior in most situations?

    Did the sex of your partner make a difference? How?

    What did you learn about yourself in this exercise?

5. A total class sharing after partner reflection often increases an individual's awareness of the diversity of feelings and behavioral responses, as well as providing support for one's own reactions.

⁂

SUBJECT: *"A Sexual Act Should Be ..."*

MATERIALS NEEDED:

For each person, an envelope containing slips with the 11 value positions on page 140.
In Procedure Alternative II, a Preference Sort Continuum (see page 143) for each person.
One sheet of paper per group.

TIME REQUIRED: 30-60 minutes.

OBJECTIVES:

To clarify various values regarding sexual choice, by means of a forced-choice situation.

To provide a springboard for discussion and interaction about sexual decisions.

RATIONALE:

A forced-choice situation makes it obligatory for people to examine the relative importance of their values and act on them in designating a choice. Many will object that they "cannot" make this choice, but if the directions are consistent and insistent, the resulting discussion will be more sharply focused and will reveal more diversity.

As with other exercises in this book, the structure involves everyone in the group, and thus makes it easier for reticent or inhibited students to participate.

TWO ALTERNATIVE PROCEDURES: For both, the students should form into groups of four to six and examine the 11 value positions below. Each statement should be printed on a slip of paper.

1. A sexual act should bring an increased capacity to trust self and others.

2. A sexual act should contribute to fun and pleasure.

3. A sexual act should increase the possibility of honesty and openness.

4. A sexual act should provide physical release.

5. A sexual act should allow complete freedom for the individual.

6. A sexual act should increase the chances of mutuality and communication in a relationship.

7. A sexual act should free a person from the constraints of society, family, tradition.

8. A sexual act should enhance the self-respect of all involved.

9. A sexual act should enable people to "do their own thing."

10. A sexual act should be based on, express and/or deepen the participants' commitment to one another.

11. A sexual act should be consistent with the religious convictions of the person involved.

PROCEDURE: Alternative I

1. Say:

"Read the 11 statements carefully. Then sort them into three piles.

"In pile Number 1, put the one slip which *best* characterizes for you what a sexual act should do or be.

"In pile Number 3, put the one slip which *least* characterizes for you what a sexual act should do or be.

"Put the other nine slips in the center pile.

"As you read and sort through the slips, remember that they refer to a *sexual act,* which may include not only heterosexual but homosexual or solo sex.

"You may find it difficult to make these choices. You may want to include two or three in pile 1 and none in pile 3. But in sexual situations, you do finally have to put yourself on the line and choose between this option and that one—rarely can you have both. Therefore, choose the *best* option for *you*—even though there may be only the slightest shade of difference between that option and another."

2. When participants have finished the sorting, suggest that they discuss their choices in their group:

"Talk now with members of your group about the choices you made. Focus especially on helping each other clarify why they chose a particular option. It is possible to serve a clarifying function without being argumentative or judgmental. Listen carefully, especially to those whose choices differ from yours. Ask for the reasoning behind the choices made."

3. When discussion seems to be on the wane, hand out one sheet of paper to each group and say:

"On this sheet of paper, one student can tabulate the choices for the group. This will give you a profile of how your group feels on these sexual values."

PROCEDURE: Alternative II

1. Introduce the exercise:

"Open your envelopes and read the 11 statements carefully. Then place them at the appropriate place, according to your thinking, on the Preference-Sort Continuum which I will now distribute to each of you. If slip Number 1 represents something that is never important to you, then place that slip at the 5 position on the continuum, and continue until you have placed all of the slips."

2. Discuss (see directions under step No. 1 of Alternative I).

3. Tabulate (see directions under step No. 3 of Alternative I).

Preference Sort:
"A Sexual Act Should Be..."

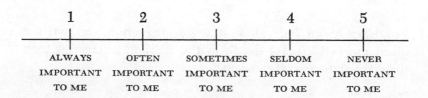

1	2	3	4	5
ALWAYS IMPORTANT TO ME	OFTEN IMPORTANT TO ME	SOMETIMES IMPORTANT TO ME	SELDOM IMPORTANT TO ME	NEVER IMPORTANT TO ME

NONMARITAL SEX

SUBJECT: *Incomplete Sentences Related to Premarital Sex*

MATERIALS NEEDED:

Sheets of paper with incomplete sentences (see page 147 for model).

TIME REQUIRED: 20-60 minutes, depending on number of sentences used and size of group.

OBJECTIVES:

To provide the structure for individuals to respond to a variety of premarital sexual issues.

To catalyze discussion about premarital sex, after some individual reflection and writing.

RATIONALE:

Provision of an individual time for reflection and writing often makes for more depth in the ensuing discussion than does spontaneous interchange.

Written responses can be "shuffled" and distributed to maintain anonymity, if the leader feels students are self-conscious about any particular response.

The sentence fragments provide some framework or content input by the leader, but allow each person to finish the sentences according to his/her own particular set of values or beliefs.

PROCEDURE:

1. Hand out sheets containing as many sentence fragments as your time and interest allow. Although 14 are listed on 147, that number is too large for productive discussion. Indicate five or six of the incomplete sentences for the students to complete.

2. Give these directions:

    "Please complete the sentences without talking to anyone else. You can add more than one phrase or sentence to the fragment if you wish."

3. When all in the group have finished, you have at least two options:

    a. Have each person in the group read his/her response to a particular sentence, then talk about all the responses.

    b. Place all the papers in the center, face down. Shuffle and redistribute the sheets to provide anonymity. Then have each person read the completion of a particular sentence fragment and state in a sentence or two what he/she feels the completion means.

Incomplete Sentences

1. When it comes to the opposite sex . . .

2. Loving someone is . . .

3. Cohabitation is . . .

4. Most people consider premarital sex as . . .

5. In a relationship, nothing is so frustrating as . . . .

6. Ten years from now, premarital sex will be . . .

7. I am most affectionate when . . .

8. The double standard is . . .

9. Premarital sex causes guilt feelings when . . .

10. Virginity is . . .

11. Promiscuity is . . .

12. If I became pregnant (or got my girlfriend pregnant) . . .

13. I see marriage as . . .

14. "Technical virginity" is . . .

SUBJECT: *Free-Association Exercise* (This is also useful for Values Clarification, Sex Roles and other topics.)

MATERIALS NEEDED:

Mimeographed outline corresponding to model on page 151.

TIME REQUIRED: 20-40 minutes.

OBJECTIVES:

To identify basic beliefs and feelings about a particular concept.

To enable individuals to reflect on their particular associations with a concept.

To provide a minimal structure for facilitating discussion.

RATIONALE:

The free-association mode of this exercise makes possible the surfacing of some perceptual dimensions which might not be revealed in a more formal approach.

Since all of the words suggested by the leader for this exercise tend to be controversial, some minimal structuring may enable people to talk about their feelings more readily. The structure of the exercise also tends to preclude the self-censoring of myths and stereotypes which often wouldn't be shared verbally in a group.

PROCEDURE:

1. Instruct students to form groups of six, and give each person a wheel-spoke sheet like the one on page 151.

2. Designate the word or words to be written in the wheel. The following are some possible pairs; one word may be written on one side of the wheel-spoke sheet, the other word on the back.

masculinity/femininity

male homosexuality/lesbianism

black sexuality/white sexuality

premarital sex/extramarital sex

But give only one word to the students before asking them to turn the paper over and write the other word. Say:

"Write in the circle the word _____. What is the first word that pops into your mind associated with _____? Jot it down on one of the lines radiating out from the circle. Jot down on the other lines any other words or phrases you associate with _____. Do it quickly without any evaluation. Make more lines if you need them."

3. When everyone has finished, give these directions:

"Now, look at what you have written, and circle the word or words that you feel are most significant. At the bottom of your sheet, elaborate on the significance to you of the circled word."

4. Wait a few minutes, and then give the next set of
    directions:

    "Now turn the paper over and write _____ in
    the circle. Free associate with that word, writing down
    the words or phrases that come to your mind. As you did
    on the first side of the sheet, work quickly: don't ponder
    and analyze; just let it flow. When you're finished, circle
    the word or words you think most significant, and enlarge
    on that significance in a sentence or two on the bottom
    of your sheet."

5. Alternate methods for group interaction:

    a. Each person read his/her own list of free-asso-
        ciation words, including the circled one, and
        give reasons for any that are questioned.

    b. One person in each group collect, shuffle, and re-
        distribute the wheel-spoke sheets. Each person
        then reads aloud the words on the sheet he/she
        now holds and comments on them. Obviously,
        the advantage of this method is that it allows
        the writers to remain anonymous.

    c. Make a group list of the significant words and
        discuss them in your group.

Free Association

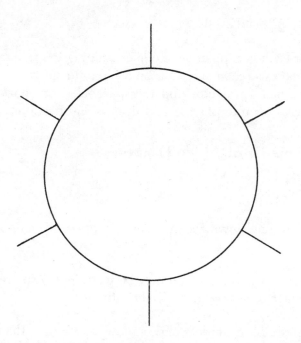

Write in the circle the word suggested by the leader.

On each spoke, write a word or phrase that comes to your mind *first* when you hear or see or think about the word. Write quickly.

Circle the words or phrases you feel are most significant.

Elaborate here on the significance and meaning to you of the circled word(s).

SUBJECT: *Premarital Role Playing Situations*

MATERIALS NEEDED:

For each group, an envelope containing the role-playing situations (each situation on a separate slip).
Overhead projector and transparencies, or charts with guides for role playing and discussion questions.

TIME REQUIRED: 1 to 2 hours.

OBJECTIVES:

To explore one's own feelings about premarital heterosexual sex.

To provide a method which may help students explore alternative ways of acting in a specific situation.

To help students understand a viewpoint other than their own by experiencing it rather than only talking about it.

RATIONALE:

Because individuals are playing a part, they are often freer to express feelings than they are in a discussion format.

Role playing gives a student an opportunity to experience situations they may have heard about, fantasized about, or feared, but never actually dealt with. This gives them a chance to practice, to explore alternatives, to discover how they really do react in such situations.

PROCEDURE:

1. Instruct students to form groups of six, with women and men in each group.

2. Distribute copies of *Tips for Role Playing* (see page 155), or read the section to the students.

3. Next, post the *Guidelines Summary* on page 157 and read it aloud. It is important to emphasize these guides to the whole class.

4. To each group, give an envelope containing the role-playing situations. (See page 158 for sample situations.) Instruct students to take the slips from the envelope and lay them face down on the table. Group members are then to pair up for the role playing. As much as possible, it is fruitful to have man-woman pairs. However, within these pairs, it is very useful to reverse roles, so that the man plays the woman's part and vice versa.

5. Give the following directions:

    "One pair volunteer to be first. Choose a slip from the center. The two of you then go away from the group and read your role-play situation. Then decide:

    a. "Which of you will play which role.

    b. "How long you will have known each other.

    c. "What your role-playing names will be.

    d. "Where the role playing will take place (in a dorm room, at home, etc.).

"Don't plan out what you will say to each other —part of the fun and learning from role playing comes from spontaneous interaction.

"Now go ahead and have a brief consultation."

6. When the pair returns, they read the slip to the group, indicate their role-playing names, how long they have known each other, etc. They then play the scene through.

7. After five to seven minutes, interrupt and indicate that they have three minutes to finish up the role play.

8. On a chart or overhead projector, post *Discussion Questions* on page 161 and suggest that the group use them as a guide to talking about the role playing. First, the players briefly discuss the situation, then they get out of their roles and join the group discussion.

9. Allow about 10 minutes for discussion; then interrupt and ask another pair to draw a slip.

10. Repeat steps 5, 6, 7, and 8 for each situation (as many as your time permits).

Tips for Role Playing

Role playing is the temporary assumption of a new identity in a "laboratory" or "practice" situation. It is important to try to *feel* like, *act* like, and *talk* like the person whose role you are playing. Be that person as completely as you are able. Take a few minutes to decide some minimal characteristics of the person you are portraying (if a description was not given to you), decide on an assumed name, and put on a name tag. Do *not* try to decide in advance what to say or do. You will learn more, and the role playing will be more real, if you react spontaneously to the situation.

Sometimes people feel hesitant to play a role for which they have no background of experience (a man playing a woman, for instance). Such persons may say, "I can't play this role . . . I've never been a woman . . . it's unreal." But unreality is precisely the reason for role playing—the opportunity to don a "new identity," without the security of familiarity. As you role play, keep in touch with your feelings.

It is generally easier to role play if you focus only on the people involved in the situation, and ignore the spectators. The observers can make it easier for you to concentrate on your role if they refrain from laughing or gestures or comments until the role playing is finished.

At the end of the role playing, it is often useful to stay in your role. Use the name you assumed for the role, and talk with the other role player(s), each of you speaking in the first person. Don't lapse into third-person references to the characters you were playing. *Stay in role.*

Other people in the group may comment about their feelings toward what happened. They are not to criticize your acting, but to talk about how they felt during the role playing.

Next, each of the role players should rejoin the group, take off his assumed name tag, and take part in a discussion of other ways the role-play situation could have been approached. At this point, you are speaking as *yourself*, not as your role.

Guidelines Summary

For role players	*For rest of group*
a. *Be* the person.	a. Don't distract the players by comments, gestures, or laughter.
b. Respond as spontaneously as you can.	b. Identify with one of the players—pretend you are in that role, and feel what he/she is feeling.
c. "Hamming" and "horseplay" are not useful.	c. Keep in the background.
d. Focus on the role player(s) and forget the rest of the group.	d. Resist being critical of the acting—think of alternative ways you might respond to that situation.

Premarital Role-Playing Situations

1. You have been having sexual intercourse with your boyfriend and have recently found out you're pregnant. Discuss your alternatives and your feelings with him.

2. You and your boyfriend have been petting heavily and you sense that intercourse will soon occur. You think he is really serious about you. You enjoy being with him and would like to go to bed with him, but you are not interested in forming a serious relationship. You don't want to hurt him. Talk with him about this situation.

3. A girl you've had coffee with a few times after class calls and asks you out for a date Friday night. You have no other plans. Talk with her on the phone. Then talk with your roommate, who has strong negative feelings about girls asking boys out.

4. A fella you've dated a few times has asked you to go away for a weekend with him and another couple. You really like him and want to go, but you are uneasy about what the weekend means and about what you mean to him. Discuss this with him.

5. You are a guy and still a virgin. You are currently dating, and seem to be falling in love with, a girl who isn't a virgin. As yet, she is unaware of your lack of experience. Talk to her about your feelings on this matter.

6. You have been going with Judy for several months. She is becoming more and more possessive and wants to have intercourse with you. You realize that you don't feel as committed to her as she seems to be to you. You want to continue to date other girls, to be a free agent, while still dating her. Discuss this with her.

7. You have just become engaged, and you feel the time has come to tell your fiancée about your previous sexual experience. This includes intercourse with two previous partners with whom you had fleeting relationships; a pregnancy resulted from one, but was terminated in abortion. Tell your fiancée what you feel is necessary.

8. You and your fiancée are both graduating from college this year. You both plan to go to graduate school, each in your own field, and have both applied to the same five schools, ranking them in order of mutual acceptability. Your fiancée is accepted for admission by the first-choice school, which happens to have the best program for her field. The only school at which both of you are accepted is your fifth choice. Discuss the situation, and what you're going to do about it. The schools are geographically far apart.

9. You have been living with a girl for the past two terms. You feel you have a good relationship and a good living arrangement. However, she has recently become very resistant to having intercourse, and finally says she will not sleep with you any more until the two of you work out a more equitable arrangement about the household tasks. She feels it is unfair that she does all the cooking,

plus the laundry for both of you, when you both are
students. You feel that your male friends would think
you were being played for a sucker if you agreed with
her. You like her and want the relationship to continue.
Initiate a discussion with her.

10. You live in an apartment with several others of your
sex. In a recent late-night bull session, the topic was
sexual experience. Everyone else spoke of their various
experiences indicating nonvirginity. You are still a virgin, and so could contribute nothing to the talk. Later,
your roommate begins to tease you about this—you
really feel out of it now. What would you say to him/
her?

11. You've transferred into a new school that is far more
conservative than your former college. After months of
searching, you've finally found some girl friends who've
agreed to let you move in with them. These people value
virginity as the hallmark of a good person. You're not
a virgin—in fact, you've recently had an abortion. Con-
fide in your roommate about this situation.

Discussion Questions

I *For Role Players*

    a.   How did you feel in the role of _____?

    b.   How did you feel about me and our interaction?

    c.   Do you think our situation is likely to improve as a result of our interaction?

II *For Group Players*

    a.   What were you feeling during the role playing?

    b.   In what other ways might this situation be approached? What alternatives can you think of?

    c.   How might this situation work out in real life?

    d.   What did you learn from this role playing?

☀   ☀   ☀

SUBJECT: *Homosexual Role-Playing Situations*

MATERIALS NEEDED:

For each group, four envelopes containing roles for each situation (see pages 167-168, 170-175).
Overhead projector and transparency, or chart, with guidelines for role playing, and discussion questions (see page 166).

TIME REQUIRED: 1 hour.

OBJECTIVES:

To explore one's own feelings about homosexuality.

To help students gain new insights and understanding about the concerns of gay people.

To help students understand a viewpoint other than their own by experiencing it, rather than only talking about it.

To identify stereotyped attitudes toward homosexuals.

RATIONALE:

Because the fear of homosexuality seems widespread, it is a topic which many find difficult to discuss, particularly in regard to one's own feelings.

Role playing, because it is a "pretend" situation, allows students to act out true feelings without having them identified as such.

By placing oneself in the role of a homosexual, a participant can identify with the life style and concerns of homosexuals, thus increasing understanding and empathy.

Through the role-play experience, participants have an opportunity to explore alternative ways of feeling and acting in a situation which involves issues related to homosexuality.

PROCEDURE:

1. Instruct the participants to form groups of six or seven. Introduce exercise:

    "Today we are going to do some role playing. Before we begin, I would like us to review some guidelines for role playing which you may find helpful."

2. Place the "Guidelines for Role Playing" transparency on the overhead projector or put up a chart, so participants can follow along as you review the guidelines. If this is the students' first role-playing experience, you may want them to read *Tips for Role Playing* (see page 155).

3. If role playing is a new experience for the group, it is often helpful to demonstrate role playing with some students who have been asked ahead of time to participate.

4. Give each group four envelopes containing the four role-playing situations involving homosexuality. The envelopes should be numbered to indicate the sequence for the role playing.

    "You have four envelopes for your group. Each envelope contains a group role-playing situation involving homosexuality. Each person will have a part in the role play. This is the setting for the first situation.

"You are all college students, living in the dorm. One of you is gay, and you have invited your lover to spend the weekend with you in your room. You've never discussed your sexual life style with your roommates before; you don't know if they have any idea that you are gay. However, you feel obliged to say something, now that you have made your weekend plans.

"Now, take envelope No. 1, and each of you draw a slip."

The role descriptions for *Role-Play Situation I* are to be found on page 167. Put each role on a separate slip of paper.

5. Resume instructions:

"Read your role description silently and reflect a few minutes on how you might feel if you were that person; try to get into that person's skin. Do this without talking to your fellow group members. Take a new name for yourself in your role and write it on the back of your slip. Wear this as your name tag. As soon as you have a feel for your roles, begin your interaction."

6. A few minutes before giving the directions for de-roling and discussion, warn the groups to finish their verbal interaction.

"Before you begin your discussion of the interaction, go around your group, and each person tell the others how you felt in your role."

7. After about five minutes, interrupt and say:

"By now, all of you should have had a chance to say how you felt in your roles. Take off your name tags, and resume your own identity.

"On the overhead [or chart] there is a list of *Discussion Questions* for you to use." (See page 169.)

8. Read the questions aloud.

9. It is important to minimize negative judgment, and to avoid evaluation of the acting quality.

10. Go through the same steps with the other role-playing situations which follow.

Alternative Procedure:

Have each group move at its own pace, with no direction from the leader after the initial remarks. If you do this, place in each envelope the directions for de-roling and the questions for focusing.

Guidelines for Role Playing

1. Try to "be" the person you are playing.

2. Get *inside* that person's feelings.

3. Make a serious effort to stay in the role; joking and horseplay undermine credibility.

Role-Play Situation I

YOU (MAN):

You have invited a lover to spend the weekend with you in your room. You tell your roommates.

ROOMMATE 1:

You are a devout Catholic, and feel homosexuality is a serious sin.

ROOMMATE 2:

You feel whatever anyone does sexually is their business, but you feel very sad that your friend has closed off lots of options.

ROOMMATE 3:

You're a psychology major, and try to "help" by giving advice and diagnosing why your roommate might be gay.

ROOMMATE 4:

You feel threatened by the knowledge that your roommate is gay. You try to reason with him, and argue him into heterosexual "good sense."

ROOMMATE 5:

You are shocked by the announcement, and outraged that a fag will be on your dorm floor.

FRIEND: You already know about your friend's gay life style. The two of you have talked some about it. You have no serious difficulties with this and still feel comfortable with him.

Discussion Questions

a. What kinds of feelings and thoughts did the different roles generate in you?

b. How might this situation work out in real life? The same way as it did here?

c. What stereotypes emerged in this discussion about homosexuality?

d. What behavior of your own did you find helpful for taking part in this interaction?

e. How did this exercise affect your own feelings about gay persons?

Role-Play Situation II

YOU (WOMAN):

You have concluded that you are gay, and want your parents to know that you are having a very satisfying sexual relationship with a woman whom you love.

MOTHER:

You feel you must have done something wrong and wonder what. You're concerned about what the neighbors will think.

FATHER:

You feel your daughter is mentally ill, and ought to see a psychiatrist.

SISTER:

You love and respect your sister, and defend her against attack.

BROTHER:

You've always noticed your sister's preference for women — you're upset and disgusted.

AUNT:

You express concern about your niece never having children, not being able to be a mother.

MOTHER OF A
FRIEND OF
GAY WOMAN:

You wonder whether your daughter has similar tendencies—you worry about her friendship with this woman.

Role-Play Situation III

Use Three or Four Pairs

YOU (MAN):   You have discovered you can love both men and women, and decide to tell the person to whom you are engaged.

LOVER (WOMAN):   You are confused and hurt, but still love him.

YOU (WOMAN):   You're engaged, but have always felt you were bisexual. You tell your fiancé you've had a homosexual affair.

LOVER (MAN):   You feel you are inadequate sexually—or she wouldn't be telling you this.

YOU (MAN):   You tell your fiancée you are bisexual, though you still want to marry her.

LOVER (WOMAN):   You react in panic—what will others think?

YOU (WOMAN):   You decide to tell your fiancé that
                      you now feel you are bisexual and
                      would like freedom to experi-
                      ment.

LOVER (MAN):   You feel betrayed.

Role-Play Situation IV

BOSS:
You have called a public hearing of company officials because a very capable employee is reputedly homosexual. This is new in the company.

YOU (MAN):
You are a very successful salesman. You are homosexual. You live alone in a beautiful apartment, and occasionally entertain there.

SUPERVISOR:
You had some homosexual contacts as a youngster, and have always feared you might be a "latent homosexual." You are angry that this salesman didn't let you know he was gay.

SECRETARY:
You overheard the salesman making a date with a man. You had never trusted him—and reported the call to the supervisor.

PERSONNEL DIRECTOR:
You hired this person, and know his outstanding ability as a salesman. You feel the company ought to ignore his sexual life style.

ASSOCIATE:

You like and respect your associate—he's the company's best salesman, and you feel that's what should count.

MEMBER, BOARD OF DIRECTORS:

You know the conservative attitude of some of the big buyers. You feel that homosexuality, if known, would cause the loss of many contracts.

MARRIAGE AND PARENTHOOD

SUBJECT: *Relationship Contract (Marriage Contract)*

MATERIALS NEEDED:

A Relationship Contract outline for each person to fill in (see page 179 for model).

TIME REQUIRED: 30-45 minutes.

OBJECTIVES:

To identify what you want in a relationship; to assess what is negotiable and what is not.

To practice defending to another person your needs and values in an ongoing contractual relationship.

To demonstrate the importance of discussing these kinds of issues before entering a contractual relationship.

RATIONALE:

Many people enter into contractual relationships without first discussing what their personal expectations and needs are.

This exercise gives persons an opportunity to engage in that discussion in a contrived setting.

Going through this process of identifying and clarifying expectations in a "pretend" situation which is not emotionally charged enables the participants to state how they feel, and what they need in a relationship without the risk of any unfortunate consequences. This may make the participants better able to do this kind of clarification when in a "real" situation.

PROCEDURE:

1. In order to legitimize the possibility of contractual relationships between members of the same sex, it might be wise to explain the exercise before having the participants form pairs. This allows individuals to choose a partner without feeling it has to be someone of the opposite sex.

2. Introduce exercise:

"Find yourself a partner, preferably someone you do not know well. Using the contract outline which I am about to distribute help each other think through what you want in any kind of continuing relationship.

"Ask questions, push, help your partner clarify his/her needs and expectations for this kind of relationship.

"As you finish your discussion on each area, I suggest that you each write down on your contract what you want in your relationship, and what is still unclear to you about that area. Then move on to the next item.

"It is important to remember that this is not a consensus exercise for the two of you. The important thing is to go through the difficult process of figuring out where you stand."

3. It is helpful to set a time limit on this exercise so the pairs will pace themselves. The length of time can vary, depending on the maturity of the group and the amount of time available. Warn the students when they have five minutes left, so they can complete their contracts if they wish to.

4. It may be helpful to come back into a total class gathering to share reactions to such questions as:

> What did you learn about yourself through this exercise?

> What kind of issues emerged as particularly important to you?

This kind of total sharing at the end of an exercise allows for a greater sharing of both diversities and commonalities.

Relationship Contract
(Marriage Contract)

NAME:

Should the wife take on the husband's last name, the husband take on the wife's name, both take a hyphenated name, both a new name, or both keep their own names?

If there are children, what will their surname be?

BIRTH CONTROL:

What kind?

Whose responsibility?

HOUSEHOLD DUTIES:

Who does what?

LEISURE TIME:

Should evenings and weekends be spent together?

Who decides what to do?

Should vacations be spent together?

with children?

separate?

LIVING ARRANGEMENTS:

Where will the couple live?

What kind of privacy do you want?

Shared bedroom?

Do you want to live with others?

What will you and your partner do if you want to live in different places because of jobs, or for any other reason?

MONEY:

Will both partners be wage earners?

If so, will you pool your income?

Each keep own salary?

Share equally the cost of living expenses and keep the remainder for yourselves?

SEXUAL RIGHTS:

Commitment to monogamy?

Who initiates sex?

Is either partner free not to respond?

CHILDREN:

How many?

When?

Adopt?

Who will take primary responsibility for raising the children?

Will one partner have to quit a job?

OTHER RELATIONSHIPS:

Are you and your partner free to make relationships with other people?

With those of the same sex?

With those of the opposite sex?

What is to be the extent of these relationships?

Do you include each other in these relationships?

※   ※   ※

SUBJECT: *Role Play—Parental Attitudes Toward Sexual Behavior*

MATERIALS NEEDED:

Chart listing discussion questions, or overhead projector and transparency with that information.

TIME REQUIRED: 10-15 minutes for each situation.

OBJECTIVES:

To determine whether one's attitudes toward sexual behavior change when one is in the role of a parent.

To explore and share alternative ways one might respond to children.

RATIONALE:

Research and experience seem to indicate that the liberal attitudes toward sex expressed by young people often are in sharp contrast to what their attitudes would be as parents. This is demonstrated by their responses when they place themselves in a parenting role and respond to specific hypothetical situations. This exercise is designed to make individuals aware of that inconsistency.

Usually, the exploration of options and alternatives stimulates new ideas, and triggers a rethinking of customary responses.

PROCEDURE:

1. Instruct the students to form groups of six.

2. Introduce the exercise:

    "A social scientist named Robert Bell* has done some research which indicates that parent-child conflict about sexual values grows out of the fact that parents, because of their role of responsibility, tend to define appropriate sexual behavior differently for themselves than for their children.

    "Today, you will have the chance to check out whether your attitudes toward sexual behavior change when you are in the role of a parent."

3. Review with students the rationale and guidelines for role playing, as they seem appropriate (see pages 155-157).

4. Continue with directions:

    "I will set the stage for a situation to which one of you will respond. Then, the other five in the group will discuss their reactions and feelings.

    "On this chart (transparency) is a list of discussion questions for your group to use, after the initial responder has completed his/her role play. I will leave it up for you to refer to."

5. Post *Discussion Questions* on page 185.

---

*Bell, Robert, "Parent-Child Conflict in Sexual Values," *The Journal of Social Issues*, April 1966, pp. 34-45.

6.   Continue:

"Before I read each situation, we will need one person in each group to volunteer to be the initial responder. The responder's job is to pretend that he/she actually comes in on the situation and responds at once to what he/she see, as if he/she were really there.

"Role playing does involve some risk because you are being spontaneous, but it is a marvelous opportunity to practice, so that if and when the situation really does occur, you will be better able to respond.

"When the responder has finished his/her role play, then other group members may share what their initial responses would have been. Use the questions on the chart to guide your discussion."

7.   Read *Role-Play Situations*, as appropriate, on pages 186-190.

Discussion Questions

a. What are some other responses one could make in this situation?
   What might one say or do now? Later?

b. Does what you would like to do match how you feel now about the role-play situation?
   How do the actions you'd like to make differ from your feelings?

c. Do you find yourself being less "liberal" when people younger than you are involved?

d. How do you think the child might feel?

Parenting Role-Play Situations

Situation I

"The first situation involves two boys, age 10. You, the responder, are an older brother or sister. One person in each group volunteer to play that role."

Pause to allow volunteers to come forward.

"Okay, let's begin, older brother or sister. Respond spontaneously, as if it's really happening.

"You come home unexpectedly one afternoon about four' o'clock. You go into your room which you share with your brother and find him and the neighbor kid naked and engaged in sex play. What will you say or do now? What will you say or do later?"

Situation II

"This situation involves a 13- or 14-year-old boy. Someone in each group volunteer to respond to your younger brother in the following situation:

"Your brother has moved into your room now that you're away at college, but your books and old personal things are still there. Your brother has grown fast this past year, and is physically very mature for his age. One weekend, you catch a ride home and arrive late in the afternoon, unannounced. You go into your old room, not realizing that your brother is in the adjoining bathroom. You see that he is masturbating. What do you say or do now? Later?"

Situation III

"The person who responds this time will be interacting with a 14-year-old sister. Who is willing to play this role? After you respond to your younger sister, think about what values you are communicating to her through your response.

"One weekend your parents are away and they have asked you to come home from college because your younger sister Karen will be there alone. She and your parents don't have a very good relationship, and you know they never talk about anything personal.

"You go to bed quite early, and Karen says that her boyfriend, Chuck, is coming over to watch TV, if that's okay. Much later, you wake up and go to the kitchen for a drink. As you pass the living room, where the TV is going full blast, you see Karen and Chuck standing naked, caressing each other.

"Karen hears your footsteps, but neither of you say anything, and you go back to your room. The next morning, you are having breakfast alone when she joins you. She avoids meeting your eye, and is obviously feeling very uncomfortable. What can you say or do?"

Situation IV

"Now let's do a future projection. It is 10 years from now. You are married and have children. One person in each group volunteer to respond first.

"You and your family have recently moved into this conservative neighborhood. One Saturday morning, your five-year-old girl is playing with a little boy from down the street. You look out the window and see they have taken their pants off and are touching and exploring each other's genitals. What will you say or do? How do you feel?"

Situation V

"We need a volunteer in each group to be the parent of a boy about 12 years old. This is the situation:

"Your son has one friend with whom he is inseparable. On weekends, your son either spends the night with Bill, or Bill is at your house. They do their homework together on school nights. They seem to like each other very much, and you feel good about their friendship.

"On more than one occasion you have seen them sleeping in the same bed, although there are twin beds in the room. You could think of no good reason to question this until today, when you found them naked and embracing each other. What will you say or do now? Later? How do you feel?"

Situations Appropriate
for Parent Groups

Situation I

"Your 21-year-old son who is a junior at college comes home unexpectedly, looking terrible. You can tell the minute he walks in the house that something is wrong. He goes to his room, and says he doesn't want to talk—he just needs to be alone and think. After several hours, you go to his room and indicate your concern, and your willingness to listen if he would like to talk.

"After a long silence, he blurts out that his girlfriend at school is pregnant, and when she went to take her pregnancy test, the lab found out she also has gonorrhea.

"What would you say or do?"

Situation II

"Your daughter is a doctor—a pediatrician. She has established a very good and innovative practice in the town where her husband is an executive in a large firm. She has just received an invitation to teach at the Harvard Medical School, and he has been asked to head up the Chicago office of his company. She is very committed to medicine, and feels it is a very important thing for a woman to be a physician. She had many obstacles to overcome in the process. She is also committed to her marriage, and she and her husband have a very egalitarian relationship. She comes to ask your advice. What will you do or say?"

Situation III

"Your 15-year-old daughter has been going out with a 19-year-old fellow, much against your better judgment. One day you discover her leaving her bedroom with an old pack of birth-control pills which you had forgotten to throw away when you switched to a different formula. What do you say or do?"

☀   ☀   ☀

SUBJECT: *Issues in the Marital Relationship—Role Play*

MATERIALS NEEDED:

Chart or transparency of:
Guidelines Summary (page 157).
Discussion Questions (page 160).

TIME REQUIRED: Variable, depending on number of situations used.

OBJECTIVES:

To increase awareness of some of the issues which may emerge in a marital relationship.

To explore feelings about issues related to marriage, and the options available for resolving these issues.

RATIONALE:

The assumption behind this exercise is that individuals who have explored their own feelings and behavior in a practice situation are usually better able to respond constructively when a similar situation occurs in real life.

A group is able to generate many more options for ways of resolving a problem than one person can generate alone. This experience demonstrates to the group members the values of using others for resources in the problem-solving process. It also increases an individual's awareness of the variety of options available.

PROCEDURE:

1. Instruct the participants to form groups of six, with men and women in each group. Review with them the rationale and guidelines for role playing, as these seem appropriate. Post *Guidelines Summary* and *Discussion Questions* (see pages 157 and 160).

2. Introduce the exercise:

    "We are going to role play. All of the situations will be those which might arise in a marriage. Before I read the situations, we need two volunteers to play the roles."
    Pause to allow volunteers to come forward.
    "After I finish reading the situation, you two respond as if it had just occurred to you. Forget about the rest of your group, and pretend you and your partner are alone together."

3. Warn the group members when their time is almost up. Do this for the role-playing situation and for the discussion period following each situation.

Marital-Relationship Role Plays

Situation I

"You have been married for three or four years. You and your spouse have an agreement that relationships with other people, including sexual ones, are O.K. with both of you. You care very deeply for each other, and have both decided to keep any outside relationships private—just have the liaisons and enjoy them, but not tell your spouse. Then one day you get a letter from your best friend telling you that your spouse is having an affair with another friend. You are reading the letter when your spouse comes in."

Situation II

"You discover you are pregnant and you do not want to have a child at this time. You tell your husband that you are going to have an abortion. He feels very strongly that you should not have an abortion."

Situation III

"You and your spouse are each working in careers that are very satisfying. One of you is offered a job in another city that would greatly enhance his/her career. How will you resolve this dilemma?"

Situation IV

"You've been in a continuing relationship with a

person now for several years. You both care a great deal for each other. You talk now and then about what it might be like to be involved in group sex—but neither of you think that it would do anything to improve your relationship. Then, one weekend, when you had planned to be away at a conference, you decide to come home early just because you are lonesome. When you walk in the house you find your partner and three other persons in various stages of undress—all embracing or touching each other."

DISCUSSION STARTERS

SUBJECT: *Discussion Starters—After Informational Films, Tapes, Lectures, Etc.*

MATERIALS NEEDED:

Paper and pencil.
Overhead projector (optional).

TIME REQUIRED: 5 minutes for completion of sentences.
10-20 minutes for discussion.

OBJECTIVES:

To provide a structure for discussion after the presentation of information.

To legitimize a focus on a person's emotional, rather than cognitive, response to the presentation.

RATIONALE:

A minimal structure, such as the use of these incomplete sentences, makes discussion easier, especially in groups in which the members are new to each other.

Writing down responses to the presentation facilitates sharing of feelings, since to some people reading one's responses seems less threatening than spontaneous discussion.

The written response gives form to the discussion. Otherwise, some persons might feel hesitant about admitting their ignorance or lack of sophistication about certain information.

PROCEDURE:

1. Instruct the students to get into groups of six before presentation of the film, lecture, whatever.

2. After the presentation, put on the overhead, or on a chart, the following sentence fragments. Instruct the students to complete the sentences.

> After seeing this film (hearing this lecture, etc.) I feel...
>
> I was surprised to find out...
>
> I am still not clear about...
>
> The thing I think I'll remember most about the presentation is...

3. Use the students' completed sentences as a springboard for discussion in your groups.

☀   ☀   ☀

SUBJECT: *Similes*

MATERIALS NEEDED: Pencils and 3 x 5 cards.

TIME REQUIRED: 20 minutes, in addition to time for film.

OBJECTIVES:

To emphasize aspects of sexuality other than anatomy.

To identify and interpret various sexual issues presented in symbolic form.

To encourage persons to invest ambiguous or abstract images with their own meanings, and to explore these meanings with others.

RATIONALE:

Since so much traditional sex education has dealt with "the facts of life," there is a need to legitimize the *feeling* aspects of sexuality.

The factual approach to sexuality emphasizes "right answers." One of the useful features of abstract and metaphorical art in the teaching of sexuality is its susceptibility to a number of interpretations. This activity encourages persons to invest the film (lecture, tape, etc.) with their own meanings and then to discover what the same event means to others. This process often leads to increased awareness of the diverse assumptions and feelings each of us brings to life's situations.

PROCEDURE:

1. Instruct the participants to form groups of six before the presentation.

2. Immediately following the presentation, pass out about twenty 3 x 5 cards to each group. Then say:

   "Each person complete the following sentence with an appropriate and vivid simile—'Sex in this film (tape, etc.) is like . . .'

   "A simile involves drawing comparisons between two unlike entities. Let your mind run free—think of as wild a comparison as you can to express the innermost sexual feelings or meaning that you perceive here.

   "Create as many similes as you can in the time allowed. Write each on a separate card."

3. NOTE TO LEADER: It may be helpful to give examples of similes to the students. Here are some examples of similes written by students at Michigan State after seeing the film *Quickie*:

   In this film, sex is like "looking through a blank book, expecting to find something and closing it, because there was nothing there."

   In this film, sex is like "bolting your dessert."

   In this film, sex is like "a duck on a pond—serene on the surface, but paddling like the devil underneath."

4. When everyone in the group has finished, ask all to lay their cards face down in the center of the group. Shuffle

them, and then ask each person to draw one or more out (depending on how many cards there are).

5. Before any similes are read, give the following directions:

"Each person will read the simile he/she has drawn. If it is the one you wrote, do not let your group know. Read one simile at a time, and allow each group member to say what the simile means personally. After all students have expressed themselves, the writer of that simile indicates what he/she intended to express and what in the film (or tape, etc.) prompted that response."

6. Instruct the group to follow the same procedure with the other similes. Give them some indication of the amount of time available for this exercise so they can pace themselves.

7. As a conclusion, it might be valuable for the group to see if there were any recurring themes in the similes. If so, this could then be shared in a total class gathering.

※　　※　　※

SUBJECT: *Choosing from a Field of Words—For Use After Films, Tapes, Lectures, Etc.*

MATERIALS NEEDED:

Mimeographed sheet filled randomly with words (see page 202 for model), or chart plus paper and pencil for each student.

TIME REQUIRED: 15-40 minutes.

OBJECTIVES:

To force a choice among a number of options.

To provide a springboard for discussion about different student perceptions of the presentation.

To expose participants to some alternative views of the presentation which might not be generated spontaneously with the group.

RATIONALE:

One of the important processes in group-centered teaching of human sexuality is the exposure of participants to a variety of options, thereby indicating to students both the range of choices and the necessity of choosing.

This activity is useful in groups where the leader wishes to raise the level of insight and perception about diversity of life styles or value options. By providing the list of words to choose from, the leader may be widening the range of vision.

When only three choices are allowed from a list of 15-25 words, participants must place priorities on their possible decisions.

Other groups may find it more productive to generate their own list of words (see next exercise).

PROCEDURE:

1. Before the presentation begins, direct the students to form groups of six.

2. After the presentation, pass out to students mimeographed sheets with words arranged randomly, as on 202 (or post the words on a chart).

3. NOTE TO LEADER: You will probably prefer to provide a different field of words, one which is more appropriate to the specific content of your presentation than the field which follows.

4. Give instructions:

   "Using the sheet in front of you, circle (or write, if the sheet is blank) the three words from the field that best describe your perception of the presentation. Trust your first inclinations and circle (or write) those words. Do this quickly."

5. Allow a few minutes for them to do this, then continue your instructions:

   "Now you are to tabulate your choices. One person in each group be the recorder and write down the choices of those in your group. Take a look at how your group tabulation comes out. You may want to talk about the most frequently recurring word choices, or the ones that were chosen least frequently. Ask people to give reasons for their choices."

Choosing from a Field of Words

Circle the three words which best express what *you* saw or heard in the film or other presentation.

intimacy

equality   exploitation

game   "lay"

impersonality

fun   casual sex

affection

aggression   relationship

sharing

irresponsibility   freedom

submitting

non-commitment

taking   spontaneity

oppression

who initiated ⎰ man
               ⎱ both
                 woman

SUBJECT: *Generating a Field of Words—To Be Used Following a Film, Tape, Lecture, Etc.*

MATERIALS NEEDED:

Pencils and paper.
Chart or overhead projector.

TIME REQUIRED: 15-30 minutes.

OBJECTIVES:

To provide a springboard for sharing perceptions about the presentation.

To legitimize multiple responses to a given presentation.

RATIONALE:

Writing down responses sometimes makes it easier for timid persons or those with a minority viewpoint to express their view. If they are expected to react spontaneously, they may contribute nothing.

Asking students to generate as many words as possible encourages the group to look at diverse responses to the presentation.

PROCEDURE: Alternative I

1. Before the presentation, instruct the participants to form groups of six.

2. After the presentation, distribute paper and pencils to each group and introduce exercise:

    "Take a sheet of paper. In the next few minutes, write down as many words as you can think of which describe what you saw or heard in the presentation. Let the words flow freely: don't take time to evaluate. Write them all over your sheet as they occur to you."

3. Instruct each person in the group to read off his/her own list. One person serve as a recorder, writing down the words and then tabulating how many times a word appears.

PROCEDURE: Alternative II

1. Before the presentation, instruct the participants to form groups of six.

2. Distribute paper and pencils, and post a chart (or project a transparency) of the three following sentence fragments:

    a. For me, the most important things in the presentation were . . .

    b. As I watched (and/or listened) I felt . . .

    c. _____ (leader tell students what word to

insert here—love, sex, homosexuality, etc.) in this presentation could best be described by the following words . . .

3. Allow a few minutes for sentence completion. Then instruct students to share what they have written with their group, and discuss.

SUMMARIZING ACTIVITIES

SUBJECT: *Matrix to Summarize and Analyze Individual's Learning*

MATERIALS NEEDED:

Mimeographed sheets with matrix (see page 209).
Pencils.

TIME REQUIRED: 25-60 minutes.

OBJECTIVES:

To identify specific events which individuals perceive as important learning occasions.

To relate three areas of learning to specific events in the individual's experience.

To summarize and pull together insights about the course.

RATIONALE:

Utilizing individual out-of-class experience as classroom material facilitates the students' integrating classroom learning with everyday life.

Four of the primary goals of the exercises in this book are: making it easier to talk about sex; heightening awareness of divergent sexual life styles; clarifying one's values; and determining whether one wants to change. This exercise helps students see to what degree these goals have been reached for them.

Personal reflection on the meanings of one's sexual experience is an all too rare occurrence. While this exercise stays at a fairly superficial level, it may provide the impetus for individuals to continue, outside the structured exercise, to reflect on their feelings about their sexual experiences.

PROCEDURE:

1. Distribute mimeographed copies of the matrix on 209.

2. Suggest that the students take 15-20 minutes to fill out the matrix.

    "Look at the three headings across the top of the sheet. Think of specific events that have happened to you, during the time you have been in this course which illustrate those headings. *Be specific.* Think of what happened; where you were; what the setting was; who was there with you. Write down a brief description in the box opposite EVENT.

    "Then, opposite ANALYSIS, write how you felt during that occurrence. And opposite LEARNINGS, write the insight that came out of the event, and what meaning that has for you."

3. As individuals finish, suggest that they pair up and talk

with the other person about what they have written and what it means to them.

4. Call the class back together and say:

"Before we break up, are there any comments or observations that any of you would like to make about this exercise?"

	EASE (OR LACK OF EASE) IN TALKING ABOUT SEX	DEALING WITH CONFLICT RELATED TO MY OWN SEXUAL LIFE STYLE OR THAT OF SOMEONE ELSE	CHANGE IN MY SEXUAL ATTITUDES OR BEHAVIOR
EVENT DESCRIBE SOMETHING THAT OCCURRED DURING THIS COURSE (OR THE LAST SIX WEEKS) WHICH ILLUSTRATES . . .			
ANALYSIS WHAT FEELINGS DID I HAVE?			
LEARNINGS WHAT CONCLUSIONS OR INSIGHTS DID I REACH?			

SUGGESTED CONTENT
RESOURCE BOOKS:

Morrison, Eleanor S., and Borosage, Vera, *Human Sexuality: Contemporary Perspectives*, National Press Books, Palo Alto, California, 1973.

McCary, James, *Human Sexuality* (paperback edition), D. Van Nostrand Company, New York, 1973.

Our Bodies, Our Selves: A Course by and for Women, The Boston Health Collective, Simon and Schuster, 1973.

Brecher, Ruth, and Brecher, Edward, *An Analysis of Human Sexual Response*, New American Library, 1966.

Hettlinger, Richard F., *Sexual Maturity*, Wadsworth Publishing Company, Belmont, California, 1970.

Bardwick, J., Douvan, E., Horner, M. A., Gutmann, D., *Feminine Personality and Conflict*, Brooks/Cole Publishing Company, Belmont, California, 1970.

Roy, Rustum, and Roy, Della, *Honest Sex, A Revolutionary Sex Ethic for Christians*, New American Library, 1968.

Katchadourian, Herant A., and Lunde, Donald T., *Fundamentals of Human Sexuality*, Holt, Rinehart & Winston, New York, 1972.

Kogan, Benjamin A., *Human Sexual Expression*, Harcourt, Brace & Jovanovich, New York, 1973.

Belliveau, Fred, and Richter, Lin, *Understanding Human Sexual Inadequacy*, Little, Brown & Company, 1970.

Brenton, Myron, *The American Male*, Fawcett Crest, 1966.

Juhasz, Anne McCreary, *Sexual Development and Behavior*, The Dorsey Press, Homewood, Illinois, 1973.

Simon, William, and Gagnon, John, *Sexual Conduct*, Aldine Publishing Co., 1973.

INDEX

INDEX

ELEANOR S. MORRISON

Eleanor S. Morrison has had much experience in human relations training. She is an instructor in the Department of Family and Child Sciences at Michigan State University, and she is also a licensed instructor in Parent Effectiveness Training. She has contributed to several professional publications.

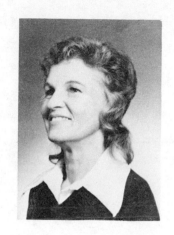

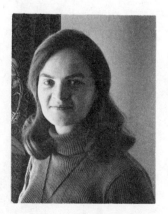

MILA UNDERHILL PRICE

Mila Underhill Price regularly designs and leads small group learning experiences on sexuality, women's awareness, death and dying, and family communication. At Michigan State University, she coordinates a Women's Resource Center, and she is the publisher of a feminist newsletter.

NOTES

NOTES

NOTES